30

7-Minute

Bodyweight

Workouts

.

.

7 Minute Training Sessions

From Anywhere

At Anytime

.

Over 100+ Exercises and 30 Workouts

Beginner Nutritional Guide

.

Yoga, Kickboxing, Strength Training, Pilates, Aerobics

By Noah Kanyo

Copyright Statement

Printed and Published in Canada

1 Yonge Street

Toronto, Ontario M5E 1W7

First Printing, 2019

ISBN 978-1-9995560-4-4

Table of Contents

About the Book   4

Identify the Fitness Goals   6

The Workout Begins Inside Your Mind   8

Bodyweight Workouts   11

Acknowledgment   72

About the Book

This book contains 30 complete bodyweight workouts that provide a holistic physical challenge in any environment without the use of equipment. Whether you are in the office, at home, at the park or in the gym, by following the workouts you can develop your body. You will no longer waste time on the commute to the gym or feel the need to plan. You will be in full control of your workout experience to maximize your time and energy.

You can schedule your workouts to match your preferred lifestyle. The workouts are designed to be 7 minutes long, but if you feel like you can push yourself further, feel free to repeat the workout. By investing 7 minutes a day into your body, you will attract most of the benefits that are derived from exercising. You will feel more energized, motivated, and will have the time to pursue other passions. A brief period of being physically active is enough to become a catalyst for a more productive and happier life.

The experience you derive from this book will differ from person to person, but the benefits derived are universally similar. Each workout is structured to target a wide variety of muscles by making use of a diverse combination of exercises. It may take some time to adjust to some of the exercises, but once you go through the motion a couple of times, it will become easier over time. If for any reason you feel uncomfortable, you are more than welcome to replace the exercise creating the discomfort or skip the workout. Once you find yourself in a routine, your body will adjust to the technical requirements, freeing your mind to push your body beyond your perceived limitations.

The workouts vary in difficulty from beginner to intermediate. It's recommended to start with a beginner workout and work your way up to more challenging training sessions and exercises. However, if you feel like you are in better shape than most people, increase the intensity to test your abilities. The workouts provided are only guidelines that help you on your way to a flexible fitness experience. You are more than welcome to experiment with the exercises creating your personalized workouts.

A bodyweight workout should consist of different physical domains to extract a variety of health benefits. Each training session should include a cardio, strength, and flexibility component. By combining these elements, the body is exposed to diverse physical triggers that target the development of power, endurance, stamina, flexibility, and agility. The variability during the training will prevent your progress from stagnating. Effectively combining these three physical components creates a holistic workout experience that ensures consistent growth.

On some days, isolating the workout to focus on one or two physical components can be helpful. Active rest can help us stay committed while continuing to make progress. By performing light cardio sessions or spending the majority of the time stretching, we create a more relaxing and joyful fitness experience. Also, we can isolate areas that require further improvement to develop a more functional body. As you become more attentive to your body, the real limitations will become apparent, allowing you to focus on physical domains that can elevate your performance.

Most workouts in this book will push you to your physical limits. These limitations are reference points to help challenge yourself. Each workout should incorporate a slight push beyond your physical boundaries while minimizing the risk of injury. Take note of each exercise that strain your muscles. Sometimes that strain will signal that the body has reached its limits, other times, it can be a sign that the risk of an injury is increasing. Be cognizant of the short time frame, because your body will share with you important details.

Identify the Fitness Goals

Each person will have a set of goals in mind before starting their fitness journey. Some people might try to lose weight, while others may want to improve their endurance and flexibility. Depending on your goal, you will find yourself favoring certain workouts. Identifying your goals will help target the training process and deliver the results you aspire to attain.

Goals come in different sizes and significance, which is why it's important to be specific on how we utilize the time for our workout. Bodyweight fitness can deliver similar results as regular gym-based training, with the added benefit of having more time available for other activities. During the creation of a goal, we will only need to attribute 10-15 minutes of physical activity to maximize the benefits of training. The time we spend exercising needs to fulfill a specific purpose. For example, if we want to lose weight, it's essential to burn as many calories as possible, within a short time frame. To burn more calories, we should focus on cardio exercises that target a wide variety of muscles. Each workout can have a different effect on our body, which is why we need to understand how a specific type of exercise affects our body.

Each physical component challenges the body in different ways to produce various benefits. Whether we focus on cardio, strength, and flexibility, the results may vary. Some of these benefits include:

Cardio:

- Higher intensity training, which produces a greater caloric burn.

- Focuses on compound exercises to trigger a wide variety of muscles.

- Raises the heart rate more rapidly and maintains elevated levels for longer. This strengthens the cardiac muscles.

Strength:

- Increased threshold for muscle development.

- Decreased tempo for better control of the body.

- Ability to isolate muscles to target specific areas.

Flexibility:

- Hold a pose for a sustained period to lengthen the muscles.

- Allows the body to be in a restful state while burning calories.

- Improves mobility and recovery.

When you identify your preferences, it will become easier to stay committed to your goals. When the mind has a clear vision of the future, it will begin to attract the appropriate pieces to fill any gaps. Once you are clear about the path you have chosen, you can structure your workouts around the physical domains that spark your interest.

The Workout Begins Inside Your Mind

Now that you have a fitness goal in mind, it's time to dive deeper into the intricacies of choosing your workout. When you select your workout, make sure to be aware of your limitations. You should try to avoid negative experiences, such as injuries and excessive stress on your body. It's best to approach your new habit with a positive experience by celebrating the completion of simple and straightforward workouts. As you become more comfortable with the process, you can increase the intensity. Start with a low-intensity workout and gradually increase the workload as your confidence increases.

Don't let everyday stress get in the way of accomplishing your goal. It's common for us to rest the body and mind when we endure daily stress. When we feel like that we have depleted our resources, it becomes more tempting to postpone the workout. Every decision to delay the training will negatively impact the development of the habit. Because the workouts are only 7 minutes long, it should be easier to stay committed. Keep in mind that exercising can lift your mood by releasing feel-good hormones. Daily stress can be unavoidable at times, but we can always find the time to workout 7 minutes.

To successfully begin the workout in our minds, we must remind ourselves of a list of relevant and encouraging reasons. In most cases, the first thing we do before we start our workout is to go through a series of questions. Generally, most questions will have an answer at the beginning, but some questions remain unanswered and become supplemented by a list of excuses. Having a set of answers ready when we have to deal with questions such as: do I have time now? Do I feel motivated? What body parts should I focus on? Starting your workout requires quick answers to these simple questions.

Below you will find a set of questions that will help prepare your mind and help you quickly answer any questions that may lead to creating excuses.

- Some key questions when you prepare for your workout are:

- Do I want to accomplish my goal?

- Is my health important to me?

- Do I need a healthy alternative to deal with my stress?

- How much time do I waste a day and could I replace some of that wasted time with a 7-minute workout?

- What is the purpose of the workout?

- When is the best time for you to workout?

- What are some of my physical strengths and areas of improvement?

- What areas of your body should become more flexible?

- What areas of your body should become stronger?

- Where do I see your fitness journey go in the next three months and one year?

After answering these questions, you will have a clear understanding of the type of answers you can use to support your goals positively. There are more questions that could be unique to your lifestyle. Every additional insight may encourage you to conduct a little more research, which will reveal a set of new questions. Once you have all answers, it will be easier to win the battle in your mind on days when you have a hard time getting started.

The beginning phase of your workout will be rigged with reasons that may prevent you from committing to a 7-minute workout. Building a habit takes repetition, and if we are inconsistent, we may break the cycle and end the journey before it really begins. Sometimes that best way to start is with a single repetition. Once we motivate ourselves to perform a single repetition, we are more likely to finish the rest of the workout. Despite all excuses, your mind may come up with; you can silence the voice by beginning with the first step.

Another way we can increase motivation comes from positive reinforcement. When we use an uplifting tone during our inner dialogue, we significantly increase the likelihood that we will act. The problem appears, when we think about fitness, while we feel tired or are in a negative state of mind, we generate a list of negative associations. Focus on resting first, before allowing more thoughts about work take root in your mind. Once you feel rested, you can use positive language to inspire yourself to get started. The more positive the language is the higher the likelihood is that you act.

As you construct a positive workout experience in your mind, you will feel the need to translate that in real life. Once you conquered the hurdles in your mind, by creating a concrete plan with a set of helpful reminders, you will feel more prepared and empowered to workout.

Bodyweight Workouts

Important Points

Workouts range from Muscle Building, Endurance, Power, Flexibility, Stamina, and More.

Each workout will take roughly 7 minutes to complete. To increase the intensity, repeat each exercise with a 10-15 second break in between activities.

Replace any exercise that may cause injury.

Once you finished all the workouts, look through all the exercises to create your own training plan.

Most importantly have fun during the process, because it can be a life-altering experience.

Name: **Core Boot Camp** | Time: **7 Minutes**

Type: **Strength** | Level: **Beginner**

Goal: **Strength, Physique** | Intensity: **40%**

① March Twists

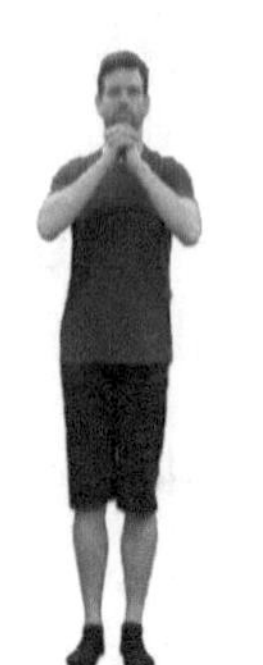
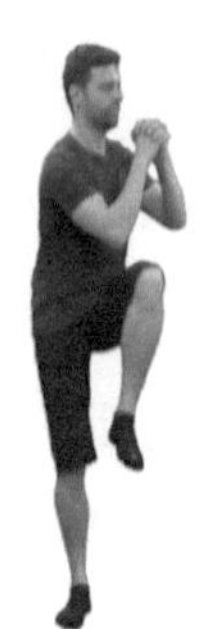

Interlock your hands in front of your face. Raise your right knee and move your opposite elbow toward the raised knee. Move back down and repeat with the other side.

60 Seconds

② Ski Lunges

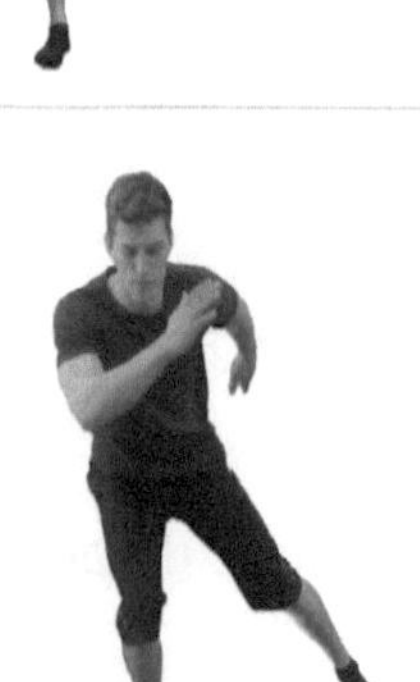

Straighten your leg to the side and swing your arms as if you were skating. Keep the leg in motion off the ground and the stationairy leg bent.

30 Seconds (per side)

③ Split Jacks

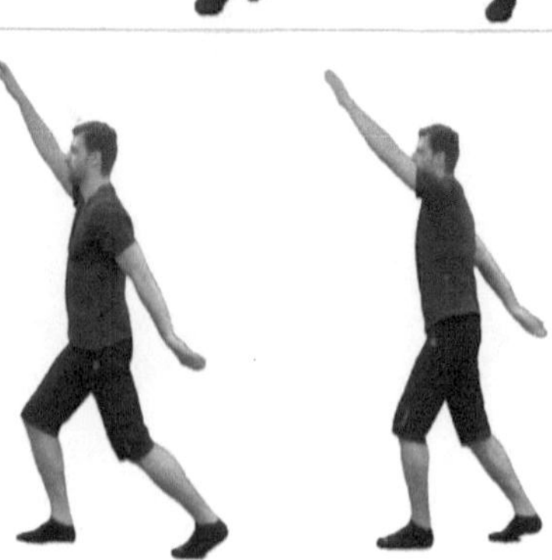

Swing one arm forward and the other back. Simultaneously switch the order of your legs and arms in midair.

60 Seconds

(4) Bicycles

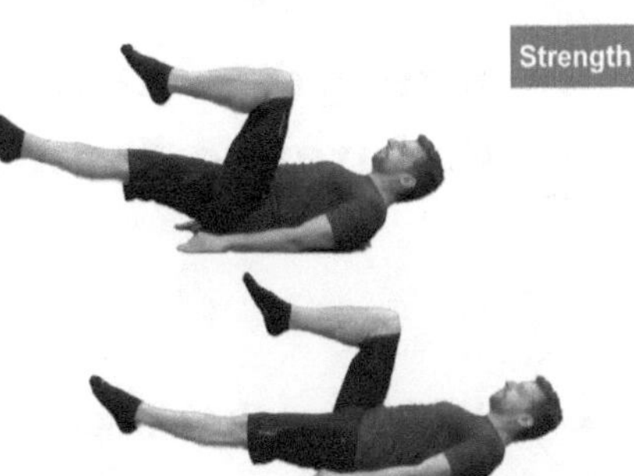

Lay on your back and lift both feet off the ground. Pull your left knee toward your chest and move it back to the starting position while simultaniously pulling the other knee toward your chest.

60 Seconds

(5) Side Plank

Lift your hips off the ground and form a straight line from your feet to your head. Clench your abs and oblique's briefly at the top position.

30 Seconds (per side)

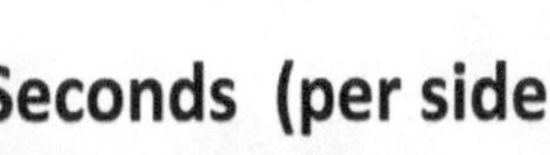

(6) Step Forwards

Start in a pushup position, slowly step forward with both legs and raise your hips while reaching toward your feet. Continue to lean forward, while stepping forward.

60 Seconds

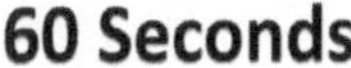

(7) Half Wipers

Lay on the ground with your knees bent and your legs lifted into the air. Move your arms to your side with your palms flat on the ground. Keep your shoulders on the ground the entire time.

60 Seconds

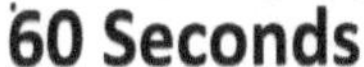

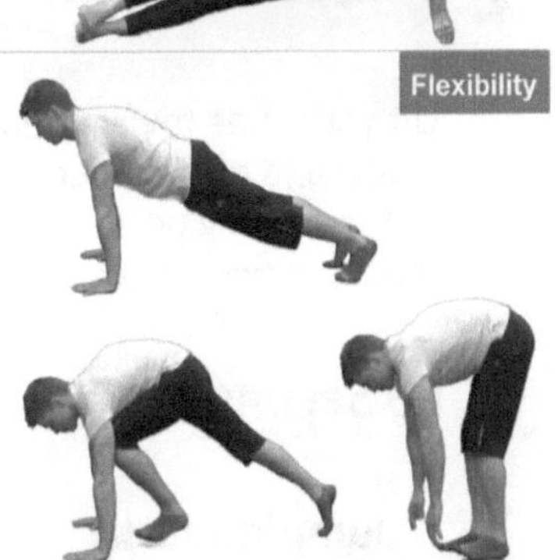

Name: **Prep Time** | Time: **7 Minutes**
Type: **Strength, Cardio** | Level: **Beginner**
Goal: **Endurance, Stamina** | Intensity: **40%**

(1) **Wide Knee Butt kicks**

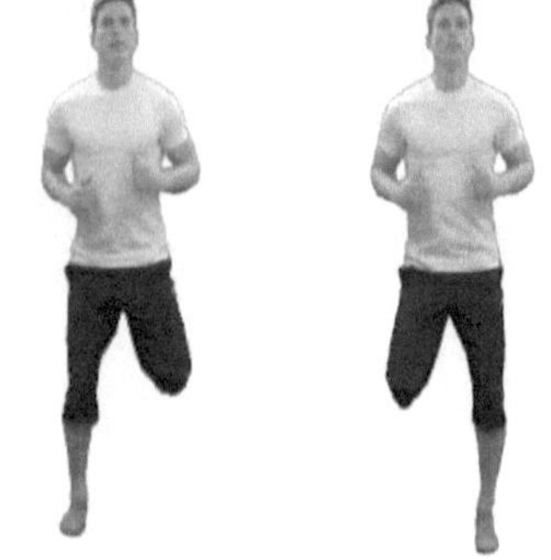

Move in one spot with your legs wider than shoulder-width apart. Lift your heels towards your glutes.

60 Seconds

(2) **Mountain Climbers**

Lift your knee toward your elbow and return your foot to the starting position to repeat with your other leg.

60 Seconds

(3) **Jumping Jacks**

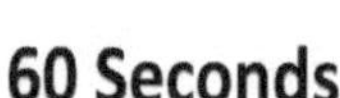

Jump into the air and simultaniously swing your arms up and spread your legs apart. Jump back up to return to the starting position.

60 Seconds

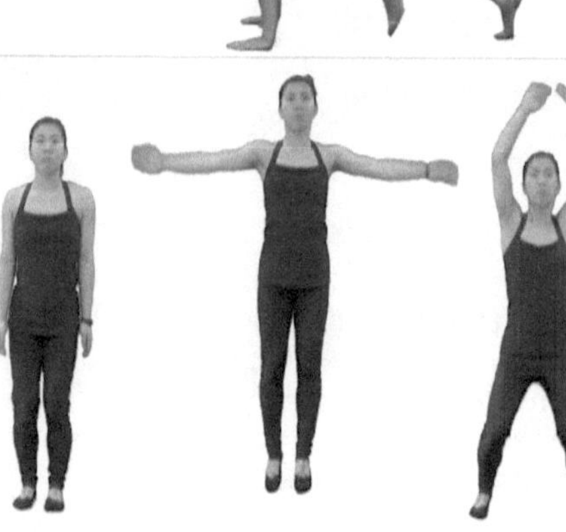

4. Back Extensions

Place your hands behind your head and simultaneously lift your pecs and legs off the ground.

10 Reps

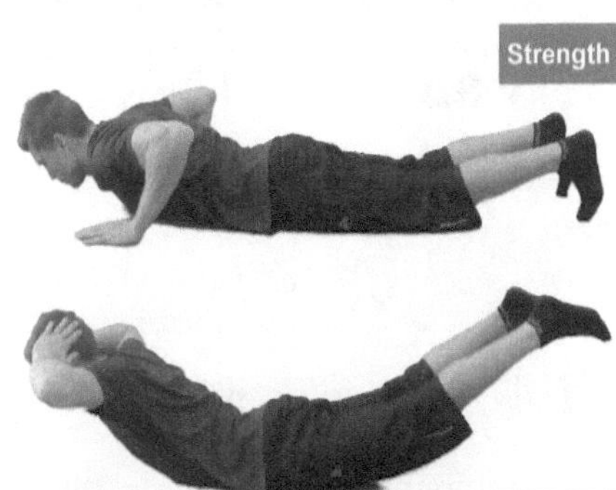

5. Side Jackknives

Lift your leg straight into the air and simultaneously lift you upper body.

2x10 Reps

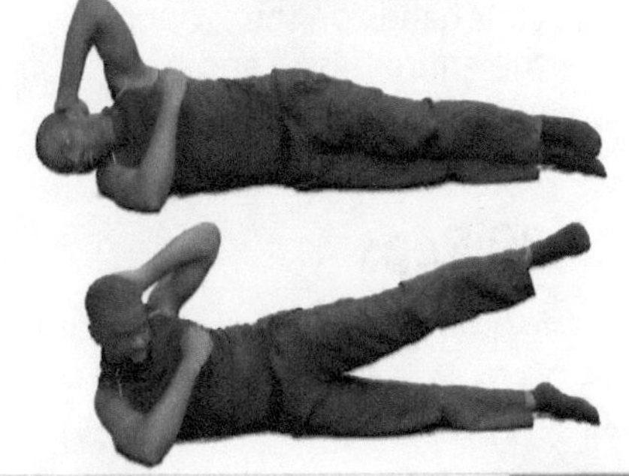

6. Child's Pose

Sit on your heals with your arms by your side. Slowly move forward with your upper body extending your arms as far as possible.

2X30 Seconds

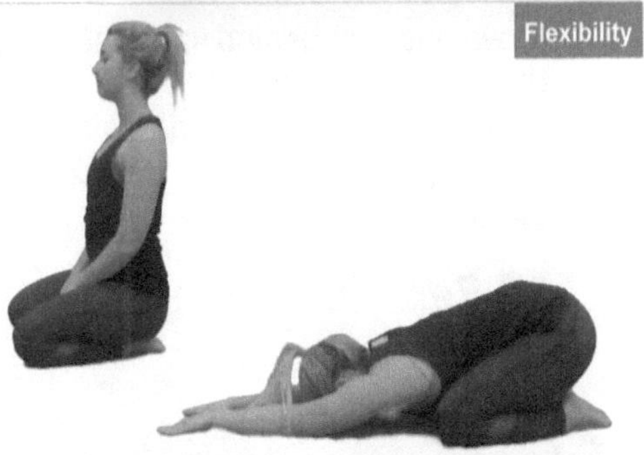

7. Standing Back Bend

Place your hands on your lower back and gently push into your lower back while opening your chest.

2x30 Seconds

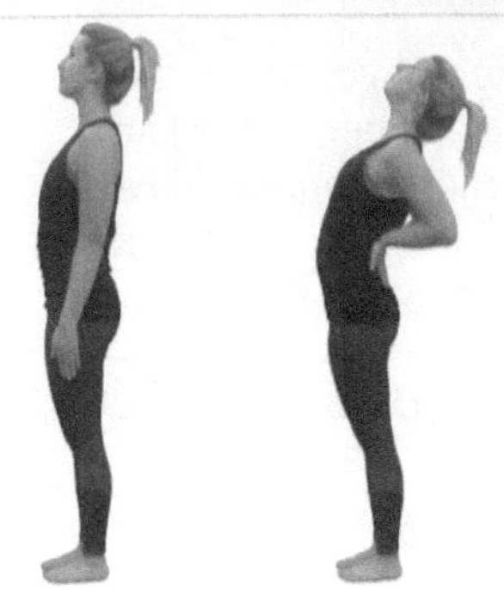

Name: **Leg Burner** | Time: **7 Minutes**

Type: **Strength** | Level: **Beginner**
Goal: **Strength, Power** | Intensity: **50%**

1. Pushup Jump-ins

Jump forward leaving
your hands on the ground
the entire time. Land
with your knees between
your arms and jump back.

20 Reps

2. Squat Step Ups

Move one arm behind your back and move
the other arm toward the foot of the bent
knee. Quickly jump up and switch your legs
touching your other foot with the
opposite hand.

10 Reps (per side)

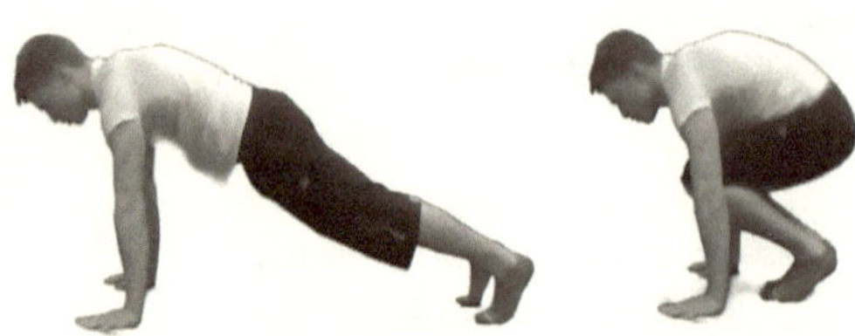

3. Lunges

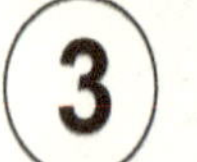

Take a large step to the
side and bend your knee
no more than 90 degrees.
Explode back to the starting
position and switch.

10 Reps (per leg)

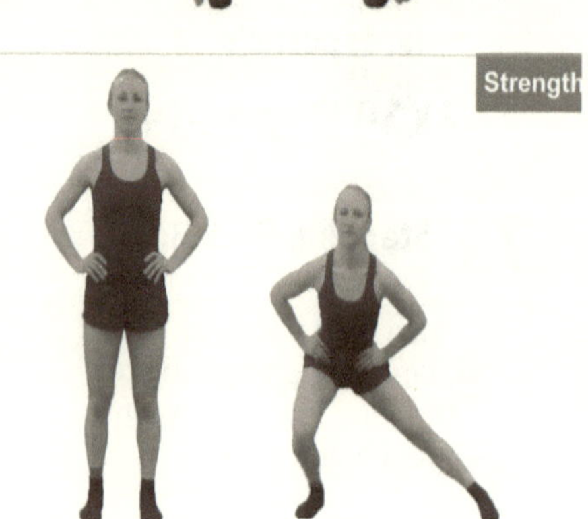

4 Beat Your Boots

Lift the glutes into the air keeping your legs as straight as possible. Lower your glutes back to the bottom, keeping your back straight.

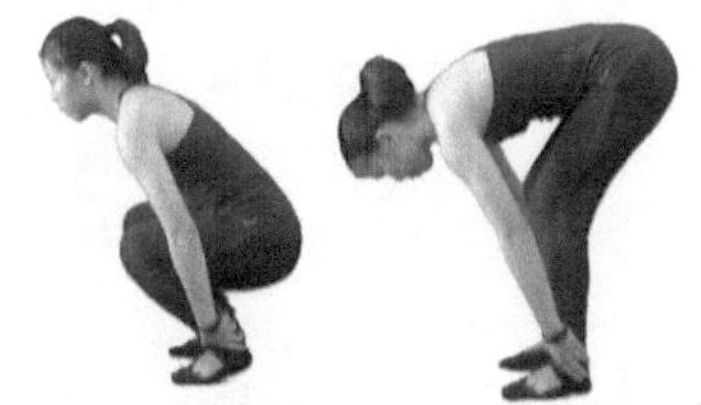

10 Reps (per side)

5 Backward Lunge

Take a step back and push off the ground with the front leg to return to the starting position.

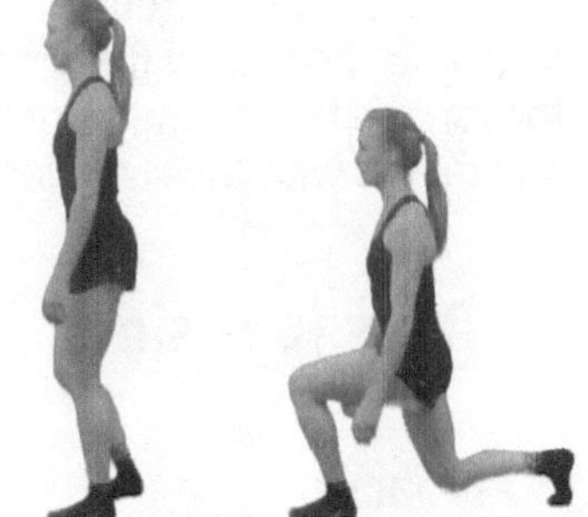

10 Reps (per leg)

6 Garland Pose (Variation)

Position your feet twice your shoulder width apart. Squat down and move the palms of your hands together. Use your elbows to push your knees outward, while keeping your back straight.

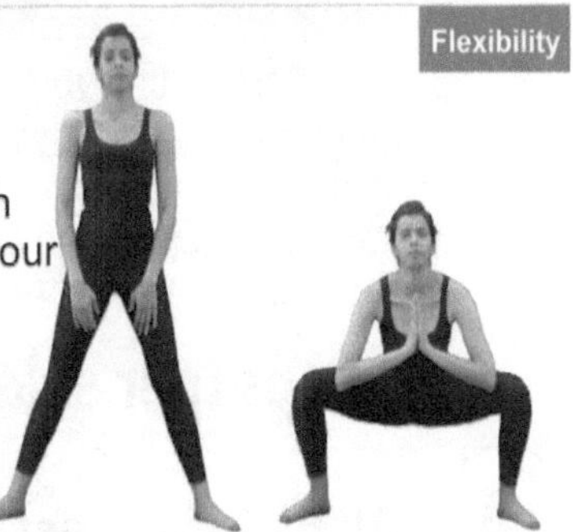

10 Reps (per side)

7 The Straddle

Sit on the floor and spread your legs apart. Slowly hinge forward from your hips and move your chest toward the floor.

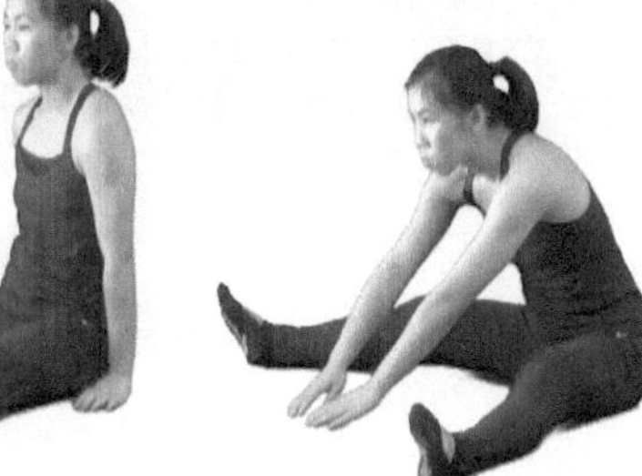

2x30 Seconds

Name: **Freedom Flame** | Time: **7 Minutes**

Type: **Strength** | Level: **Beginner**
Goal: **Strength** | Intensity: **30%**

(1) Front Kicks

Cardio

Kick with the leg in front by lifting your knee into the air and flicking the leg forward. Return to the starting position and repeat with the same foot.

10 Reps (per side)

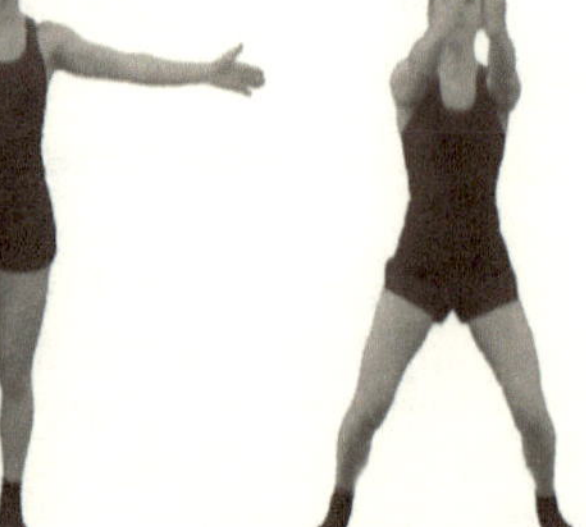

(2) Fly Jacks

Jump up spreading your legs apart, while simultaneously lifting your arms in front of your chest. Jump back up to return to the starting position and repeat the exercise.

10 Reps (per side)

(3) Air Bike Crunches

Strength

Lift both legs off the ground and begin to paddle as if you were riding a bike.

10 Reps (per side)

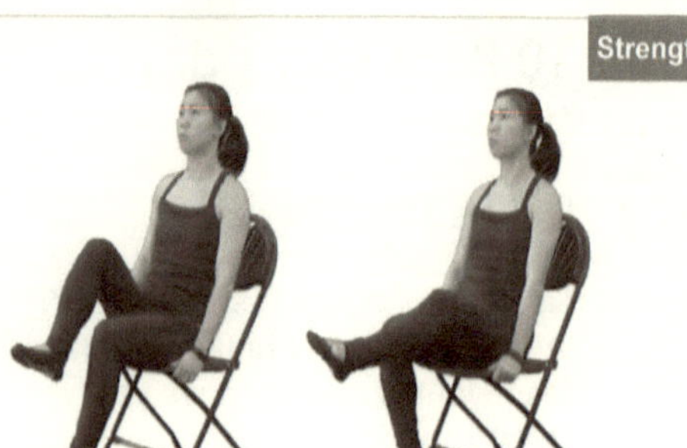

(4) Raised Arm Twists

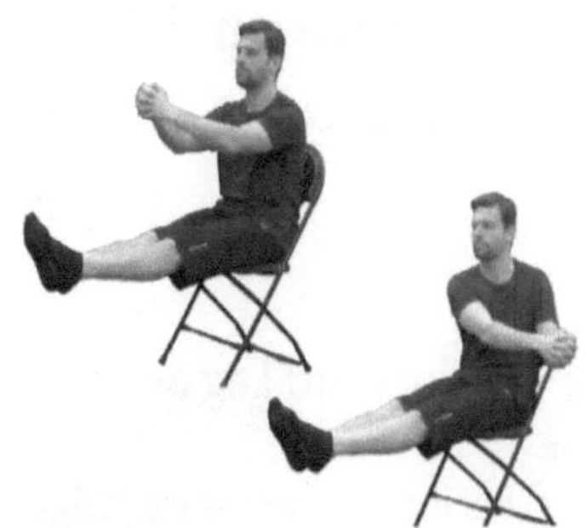

Rotate your body from side to side keepingyour legs extended in the same position. To increase the rotation of your body, lower your hands slightly during every twist.

10 Reps (per side)

(5) Two Point Box Variation

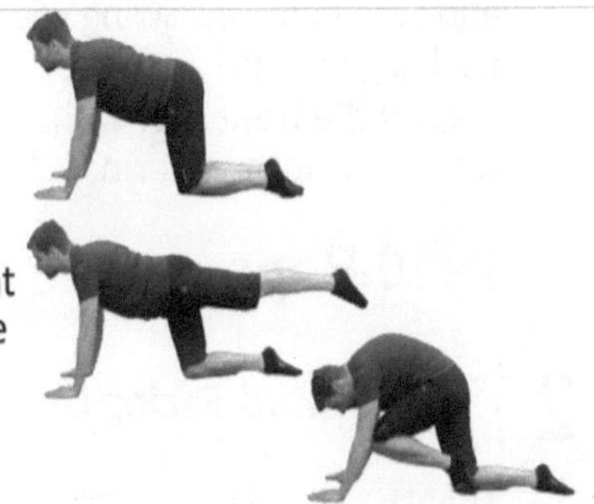

Extend one leg backward, forming a straight line from your ankle to your shoulders. Move the knee of the straight leg toward your chest and repeat on the same side.

10 Reps (per side)

(6) Reclining Knee-Hug Stretch

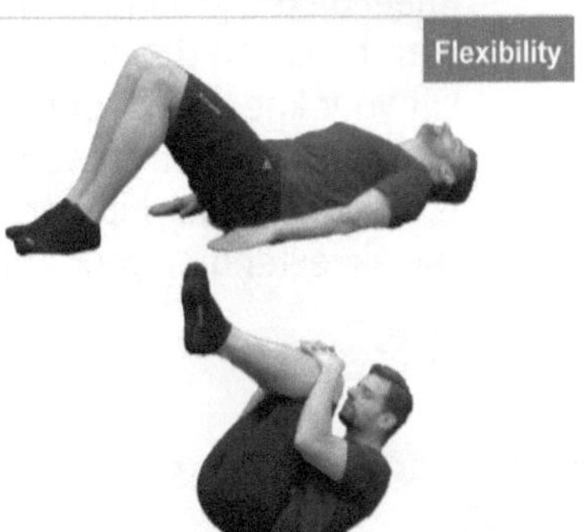

Lift your knees off the ground and wrap your arms around your knees. Gently pull your knees closer toward your pecs.

10 Reps (per side)

(7) Upper-body Rotations

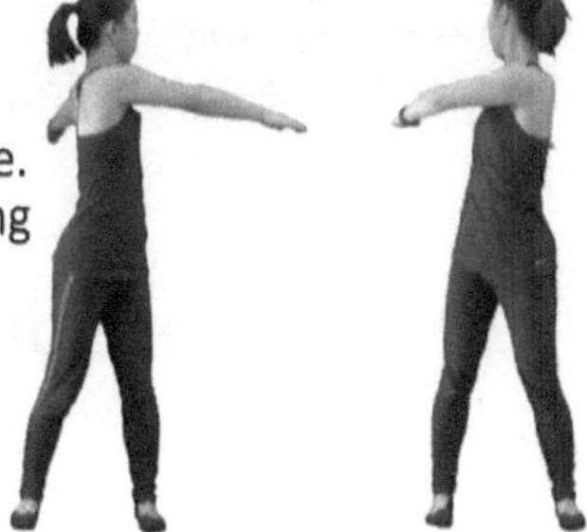

Swing your arm to the side rotating your core. Swing your arms to the opposite side, keeping your shoulders loose. Keep your feet flat on the ground during the entire movement.

10 Reps (per side)

Name: **Chest Step |** Time: **7 Minutes**

Type: **Strength |** Level: **d**
Goal: **Strength, Flexibility |** Intensity: **40%**

(1) Forward Leg Swings

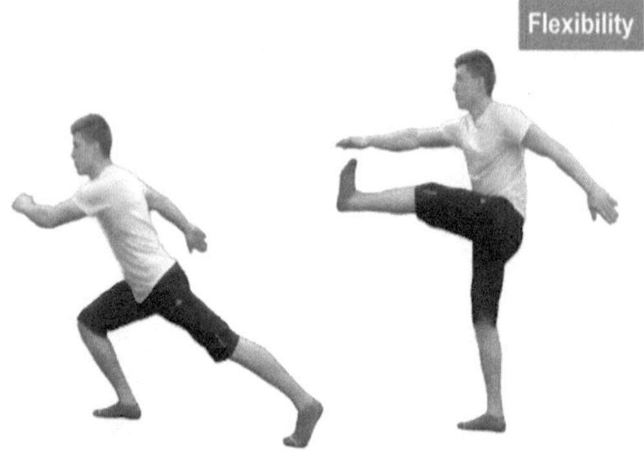

Perform a backward lunge
and stop half way. Swing your
back leg forward and reach
toward the front foot with
with your opposite arm.

2x10 Reps

(2) Downward-Facing Dog

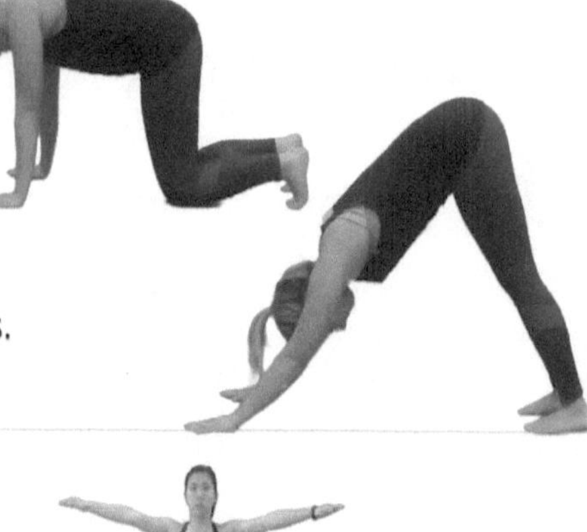

Kneel on the ground with
your hands on the floor.
Lift your knees and rotate your
body back, down, forward and look
up. Then lift your hips straight into
the air, extending your arms and legs.

5 Reps

(3) Arm Circles

Start by making small circles with your arms
and slowly progress into making the circles
bigger. Repeat going forward or switch to
backward circles.

10 Reps (per side)

 4 Modified Pushup

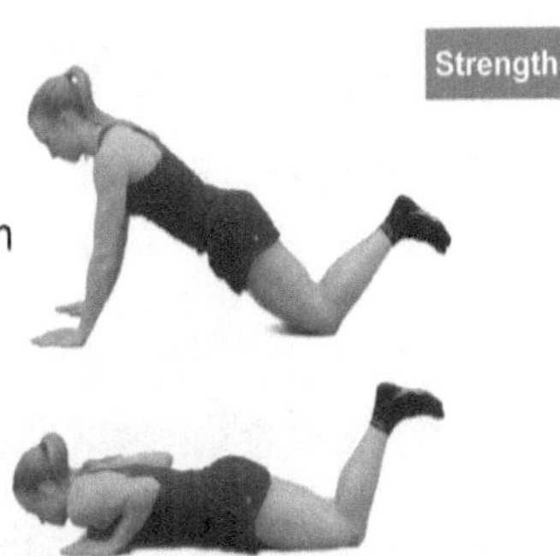

Get into a Pushup position with your knees on the ground and your feet elevated. Lower your body by bending your elbows until your face is almost touching the ground. Push yourself up to the starting position.

10 Reps (per side)

 5 S&M Push ups

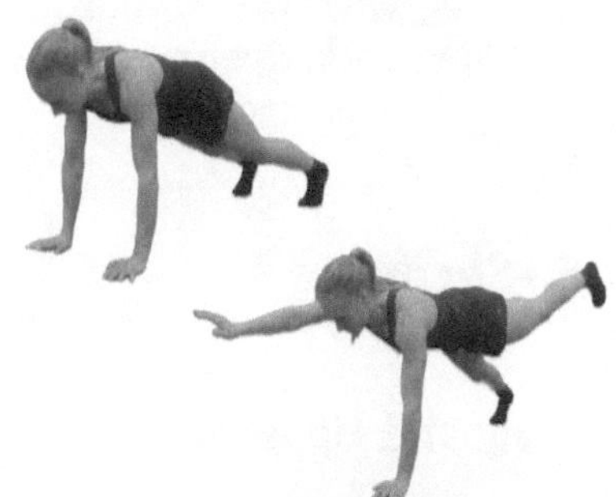

Lift one leg straight up behind you and lift the opposite arm in front of you. Form a parallel line to the ground with your raised arm and leg.

10 Reps (per side)

 6 Plank to Pushup

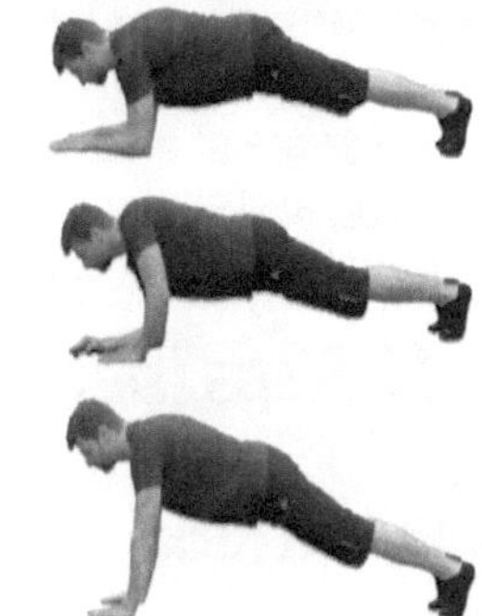

Start in a plank position with the forearms flat on the ground. Lift your arms off the ground to get into a pushup position and reverse the movement to move back into a plank to repeat the exercise.

10 Reps (per side)

 7 Lower-body Russian Twist

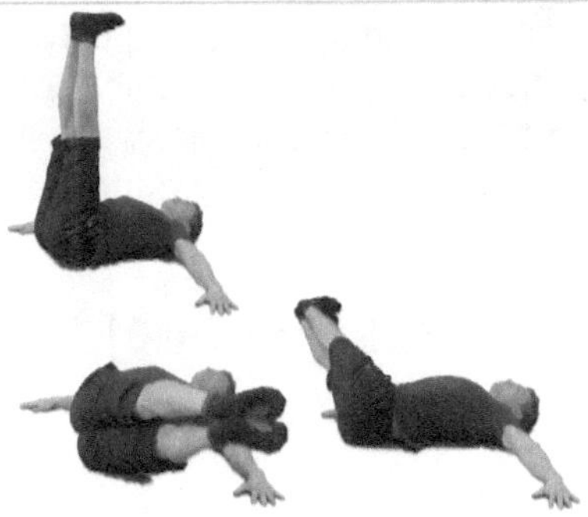

Twist your legs to the side, while keeping your shoulders on the ground. Extend your legs and use your arms to support your swings.

20 Reps

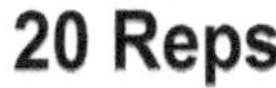

Name: **Around the World** | Time: **7 Minutes**

Type: **Strength** | Level: **Beginner**
Goal: **Endurance, Strength** | Intensity: **40%**

① Row & Lateral Steps

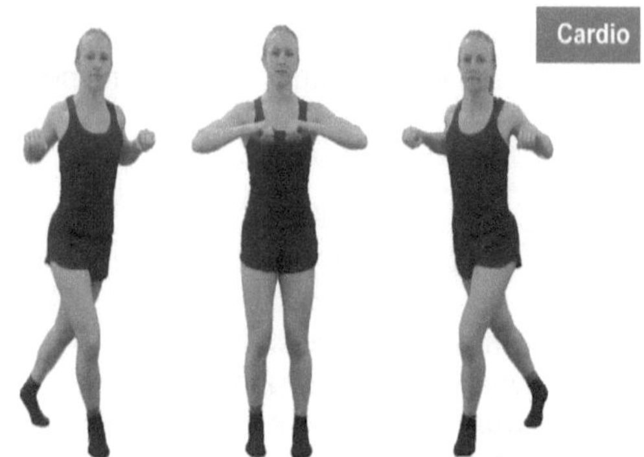

Cross one leg behind the other leg, while pulling your shoulders back. Open your chest while moving both elbows back.

60 Seconds

② Squat & Uppercut

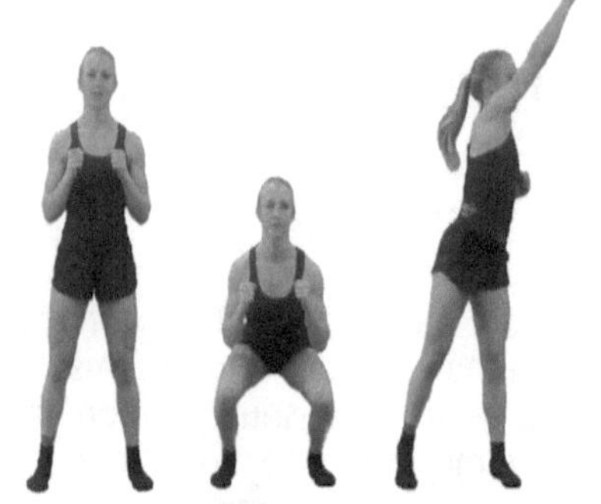

Perform a squat by moving your glutes down until your knees are at a 90 degree angle and explode upward punching to the side.

10 Reps (per side)

③ Butt Kicks

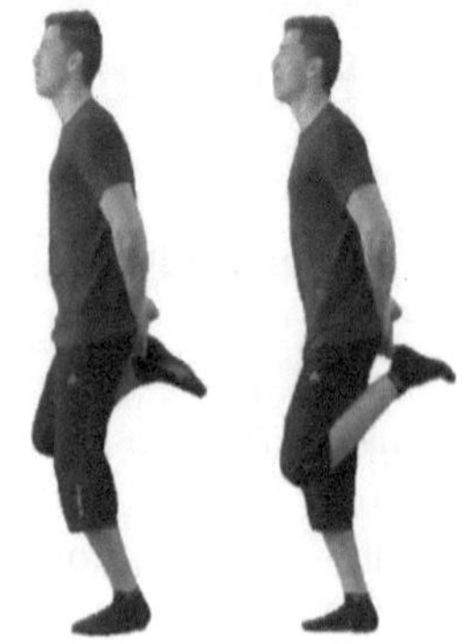

Lift your knee as high as possible, while moving your elbows behind your body. Change the legs in midair and never let both feet touch the ground at the same time..

10 Reps (per side)

4 Chair Dip

Bend your elbows and lower your glutes toward the ground. Gaze forward and keep your elbows pointing back.

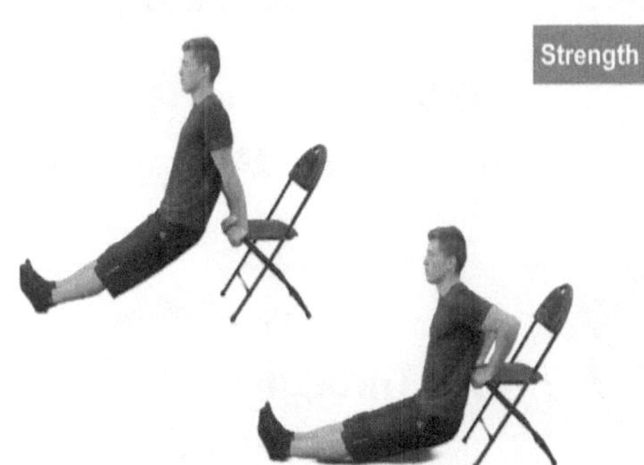

20 Reps

5 Decline Pushups

Bend your elbows, lowering your upper-body toward the ground. Just before your head touches the ground lift your body back to the starting position.

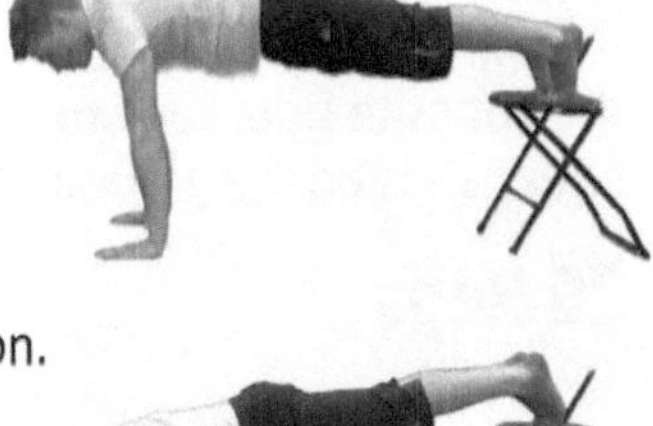

10 Reps (per side)

6 Standing Shoulder Stretch

Move one arm across your pecs and hold it in position by the elbow with the hand of your other arm. Pull your elbow toward the opposite shoulder.

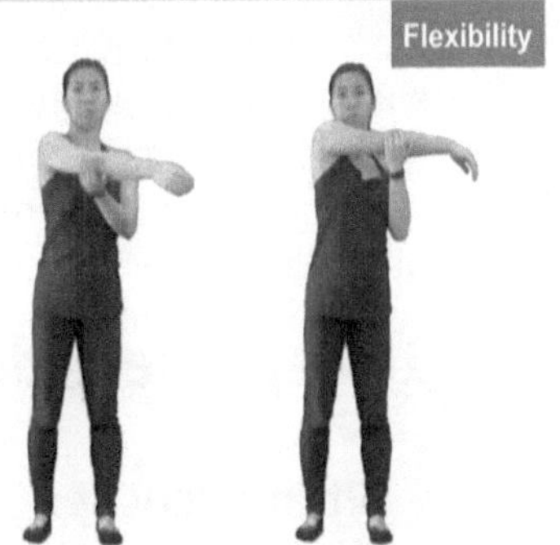

10 Reps (per side)

7 Bent-over Reach to the Sky

Rotate your torso and reach with your arm as high as possible, creating a vertical line with your arms. Pause at the top and move back to the starting position to repeat on the other side.

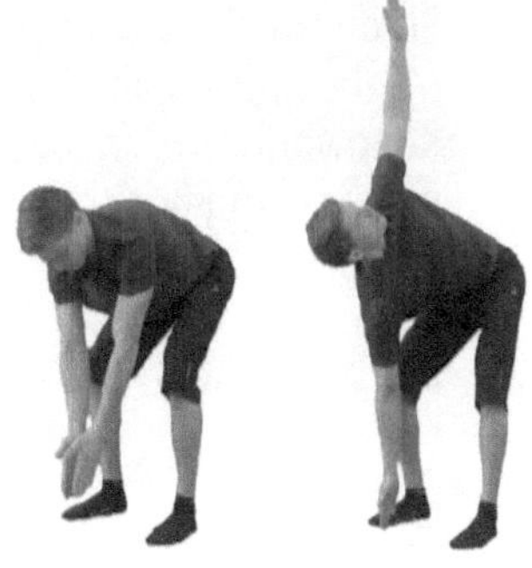

30 Seconds (per side)

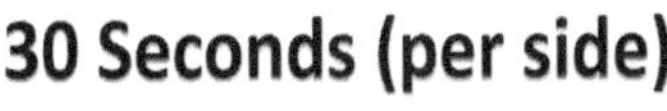

Name: **Turn 360 |** Time: **7 Minutes**

Type: **Strength | Level: Intermediate**
Goal: **Strength, Physique | Intensity: 60%**

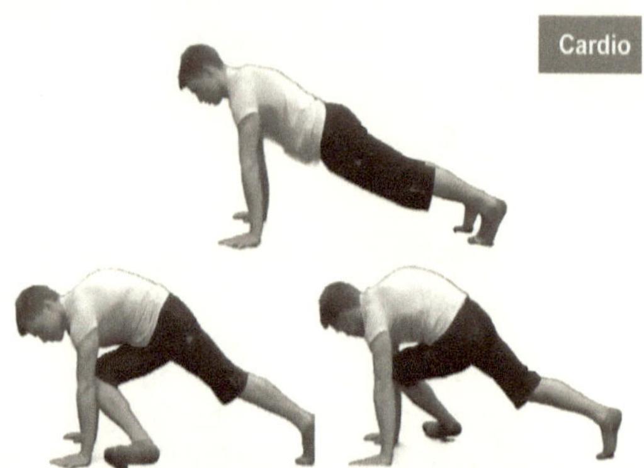

(1) Step Through

Lift your knee towards your opposite elbow and step through with your foot to the opposite side, keeping both hands on the ground.

20 Reps

(2) Squat Step Ups

Push up with both legs and raise one knee and the opposite arm halfway through standing. Lower your body back into a squat and repeat on the other side.

10 Reps (per side)

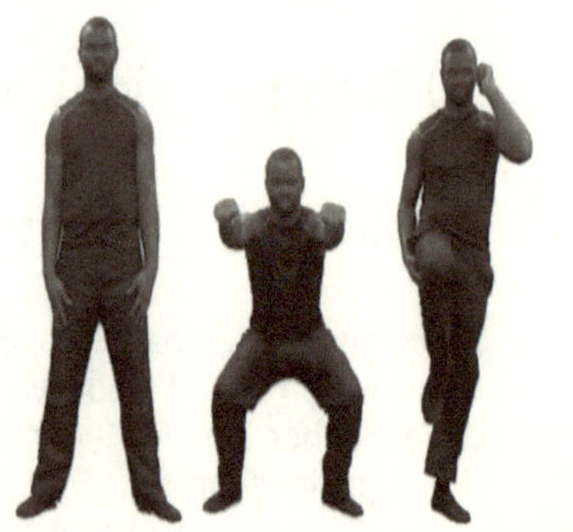

(3) Sitting Punches

Sit on the floor with your feet off the ground and knees bent. Keep your arms in a boxing position and punch with one arm at a time.

60 Seconds

 ## Hello Darlings

Raise your legs and head off the ground and keep your legs straight and your core braced. Open your legs as wide as possible without touching the ground with your feet.

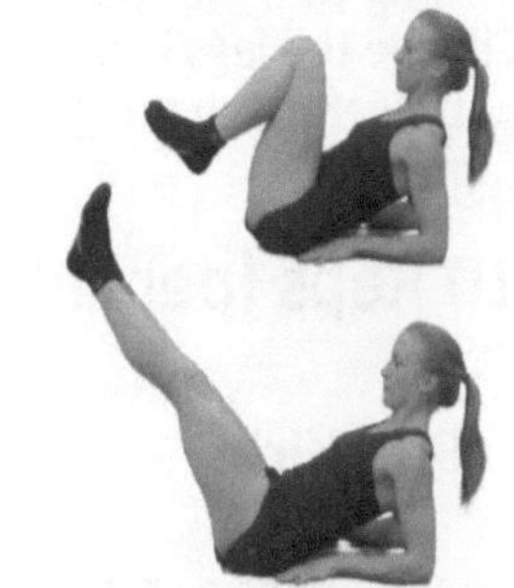

10 Reps (per side)

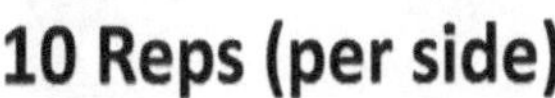

 ## Crunch Kicks

Use your forearms and elbows to support your body. Bend your knees and lift your feet off the ground. Push your legs out diagonally and pull them back to the starting position.

10 Reps (per side)

 ## One-legged Hip Extensions

Lift one leg straight into the air. Hold the top position for a couple of seconds, return to the starting position and switch sides.

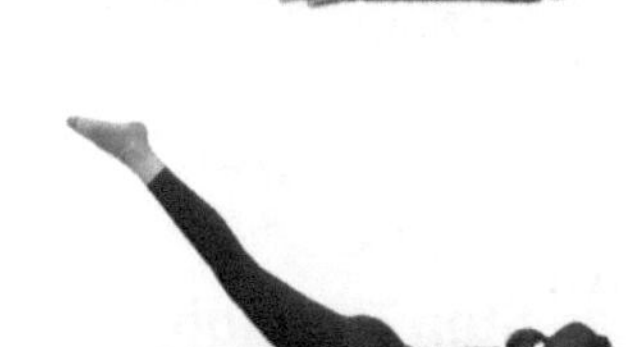

10 Reps (per side)

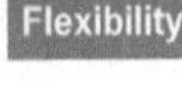

 ## Iron crosses

Lay flat on the ground and move your left leg behind your body to the opposite side. Keep both shoulders on the ground and repeat with the other foot.

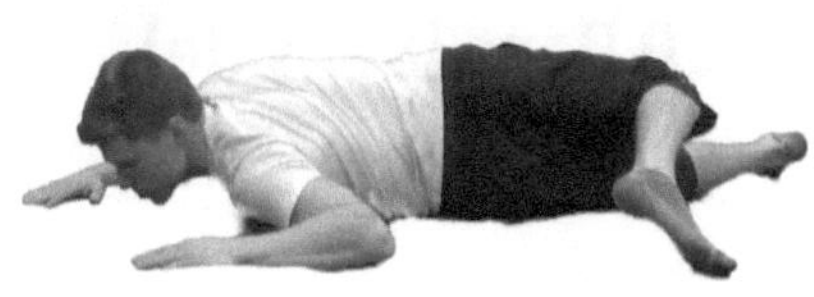

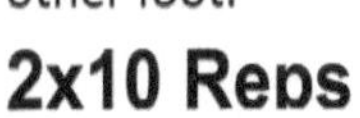 ## 2x10 Reps

Name: **Shoulder Squeeze** | Time: **7 Minutes**

Type: **Strength** | Level: **Beginner**
Goal: **Strength** | Intensity: **40%**

(1) Knee Raises

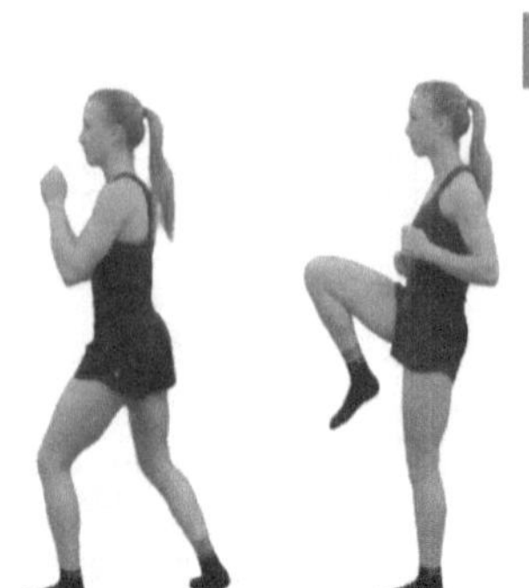

Lift your knee as high as possible, while moving your elbows behind your body. Change the legs in midair and never let both feet touch the ground at the same time..

10 Reps (per side)

(2) Butt Kicks

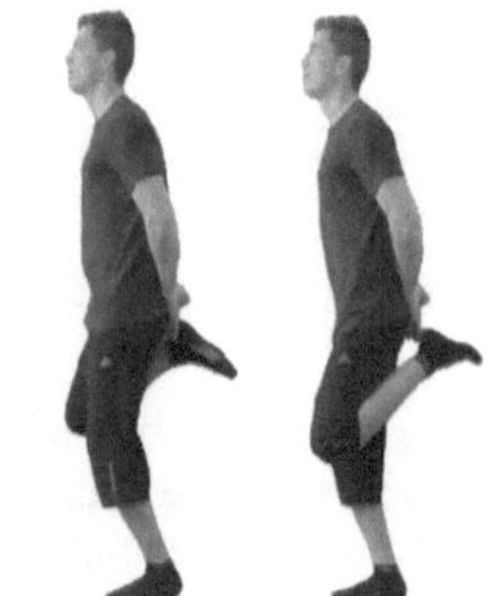

Lift your knee as high as possible, while moving your elbows behind your body. Change the legs in midair and never let both feet touch the ground at the same time..

10 Reps (per side)

(3) Step Through's

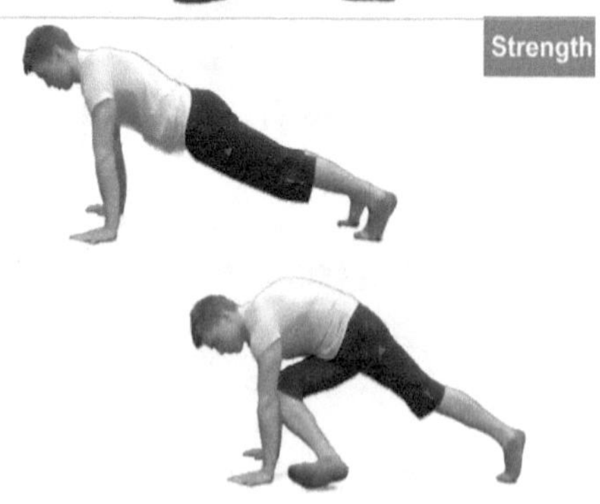

Get into a push up position. Move your knee toward the opposite elbow by lifting you hips slightly. Return to the starting position to repeat on the other side.

10 Reps (per side)

④ Inchworm

Walk with your hands forward until you are in a pushup position. Reverse the entire motion to get back to the starting position.

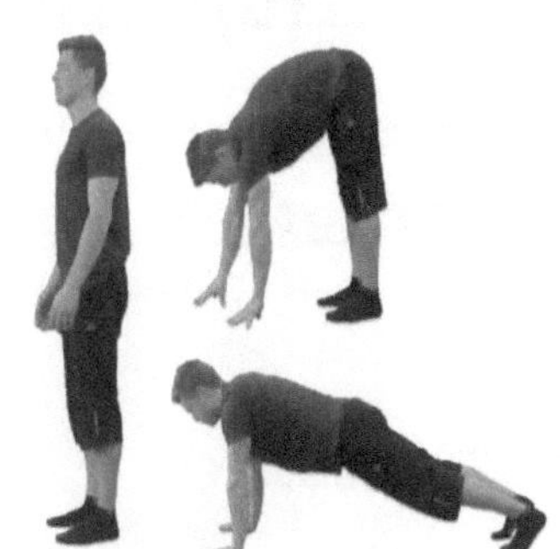

10 Reps (per side)

⑤ Reverse Pushup

Let your fingers face in the opposite direction of a regular pushup. Move your hands closer toward your hips. Slowly lower your body and stop before your face touches the ground and move back to the starting position.

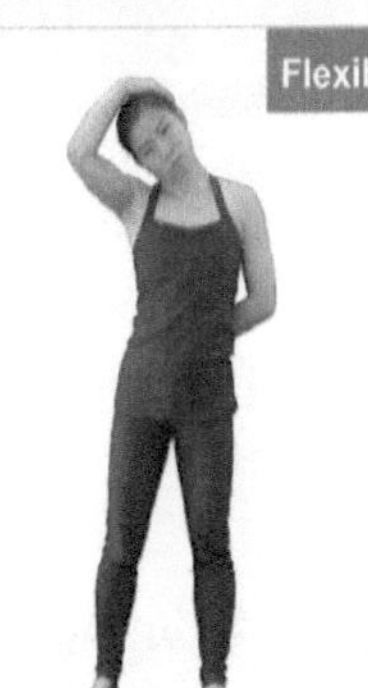

10 Reps (per side)

⑥ Standing Neck Pull

Place your hand on the opposite side of your head and pull your head toward your shoulders. Place the other arm behind your head and pull your head gently lower.

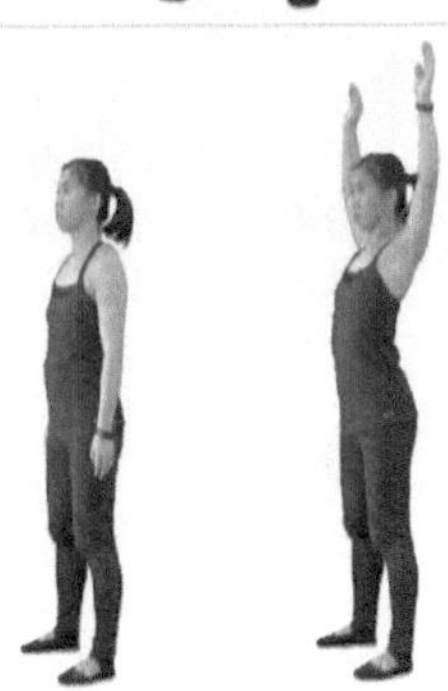

10 Reps (per side)

⑦ Dynamic Back Stretch

Swing your arms slightly back to stretch your lats. Try to swing your arms behind your head at the top position.

10 Reps (per side)

Name: **Glute Attack |** Time: **7 Minutes**

Type: **Strength | ** Level: **Beginner**
Goal: **Strength, Power |** Intensity: **30%**

1 Split Jacks

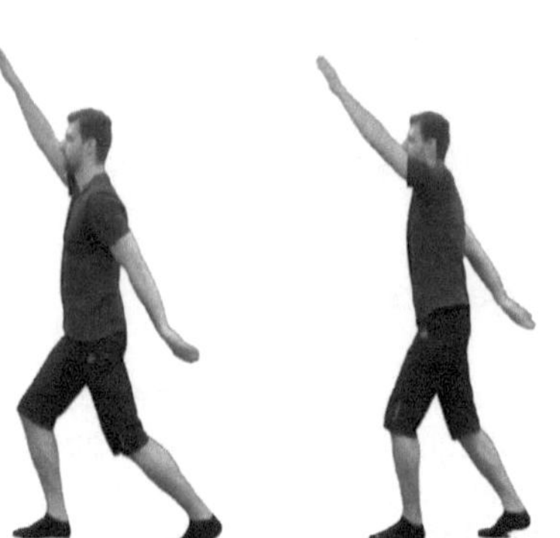

Swing one arm forward and the other back. Simultaneously switch the order of your legs and arms in midair.

60 Seconds

2 Side Jacks

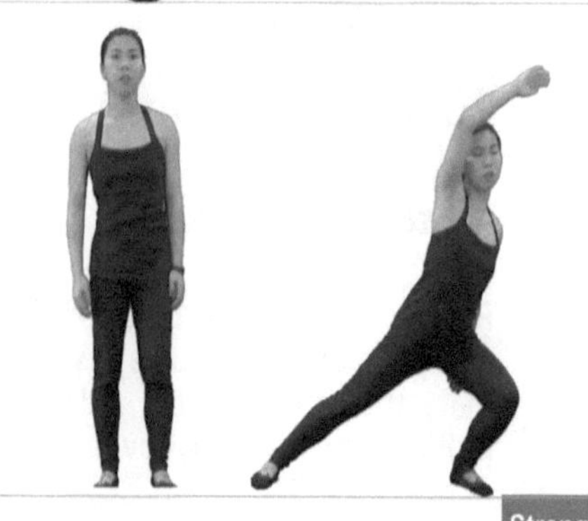

Take a big step to the side, while reaching over your head with your arm.

60 Seconds

3 Chair Squats

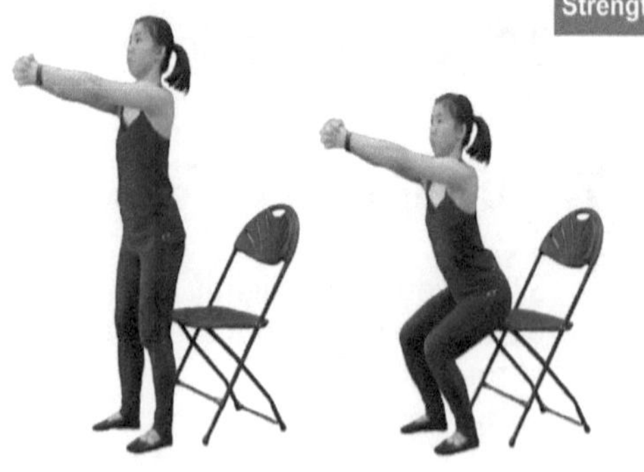

Interlock your hands and lower your hips until they begin to brush against the chair. Push your hips forward and straighten your legs.

20 Reps

 **Side Hip Raises**

Lift one leg to your side, keeping your pelvis in the same position. Hold the top position briefly and lower your leg to repeat with the same leg.

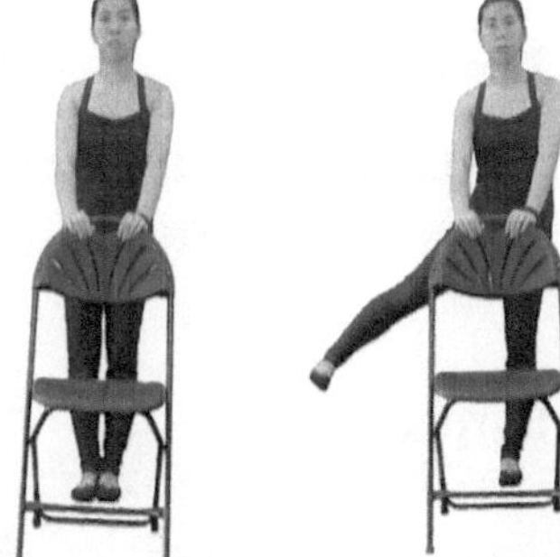

30 Reps

 **Chair Jump step-up**

Push your body up with your foot on the chair to jump into the air. Land with your opposite leg on the chair.

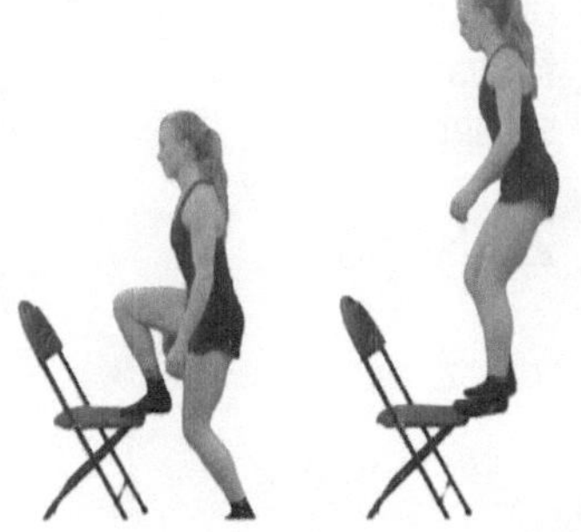

30 Reps

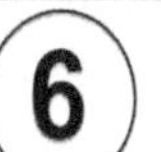 **Supine Pigeon Pose**

Rest the ankle of the other foot on your quads. Reach with your arms around the knee of the leg that is on the ground and pull it toward your pecs.

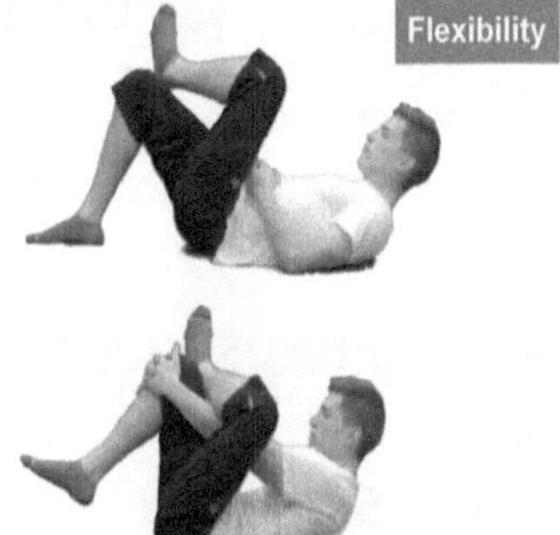

10 Reps (per side)

 **One-legged Pigeon Pose**

Position your front knee underneath your pecs, lower the hips toward the ground and straighten the back leg. Push your upper body upward with your hands and hold the position.

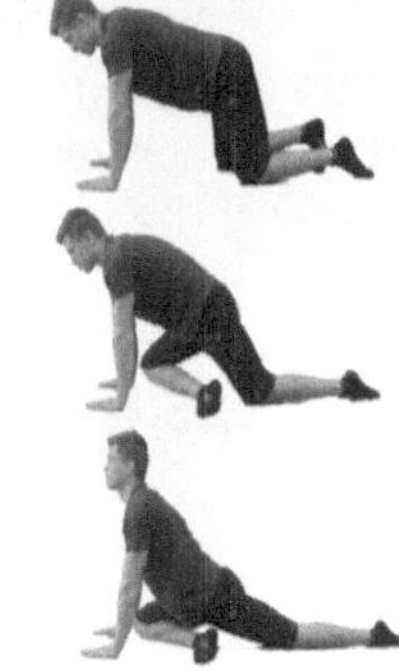

10 Reps (per side)

Name: **Extinguisher |** Time: **7 Minutes**

Type: **Strength** | Level: **Beginner**
Goal: **Strength, Stamina** | Intensity: **50%**

(1) Burpee

Squat down, perform a
pushup, pull your legs
forwards and jump
straight up.

20 Reps

(2) Ski Lunges

Straighten your leg to the
side and swing your arms
as if you were skating. Keep
the leg in motion off the ground
and the stationairy leg bent.

10 Reps (per side)

(3) Side Plank

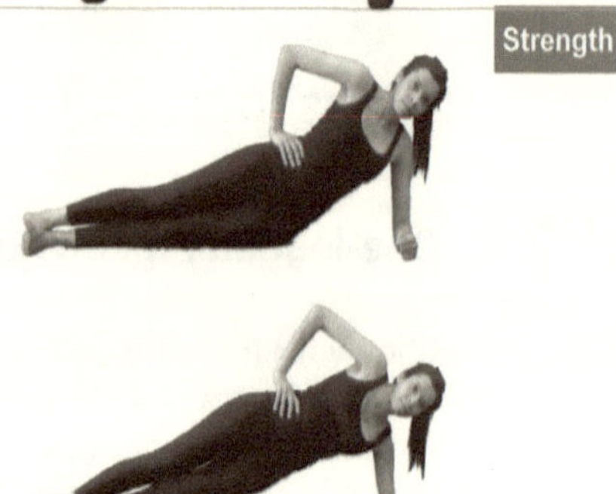

Lift your hips off the ground and form
a straight line from your feet to your
head. Clench your abs and oblique's
briefly at the top position.

10 Reps (per side)

4) Butterfly Sit-ups

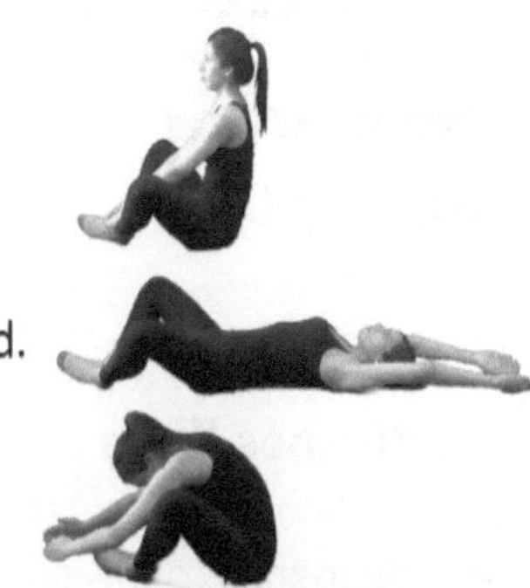

Move the soles of your feet together.
Move your upperbody toward the floor
with your hands extending over your head.
Move back up performing a sit-up.

10 Reps (per side)

5) Jack Knives

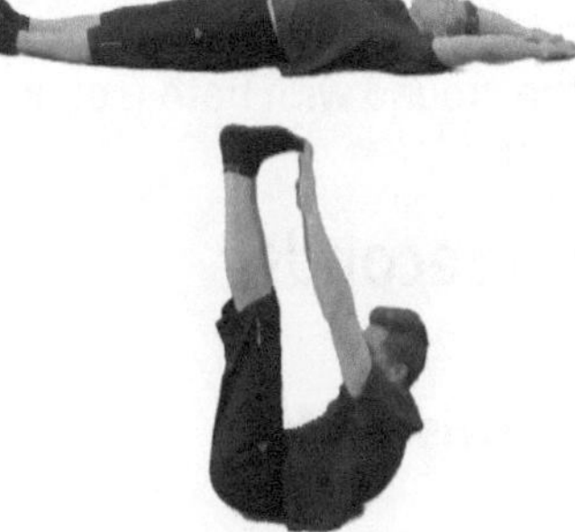

Lie flat on the ground with
your arms and legs extended.
Lift your arms and legs up,
keeping them straight the entire
time. Touch your toes at the top. .

20 Reps

Flexibility

6) Seated Butterfly

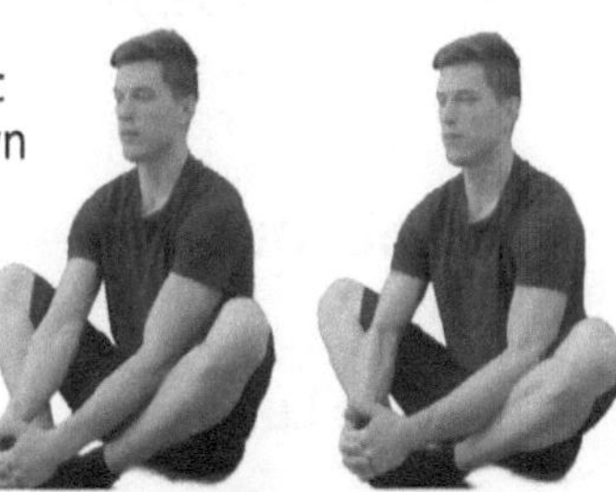

Pull the feet closer toward your groin and sit
tall. To stretch the groin, push your legs down
using your elbows.

10 Reps (per side)

7) Seated Calf Stretch

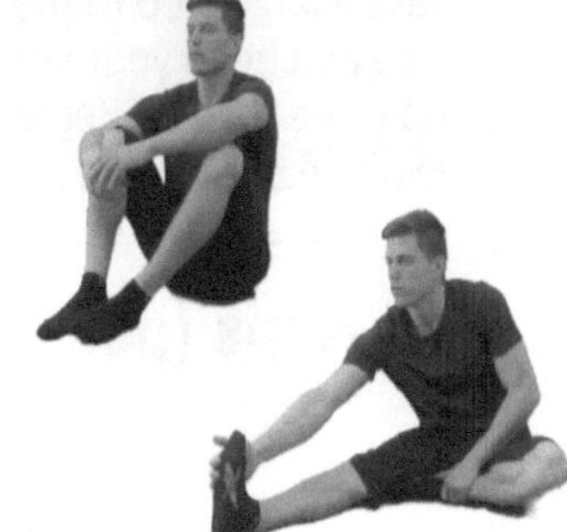

Extend one foot in front and tuck the other
foot into your groin. Reach toward the toes
and pull them back.

10 Reps (per side)

Name: **Fire Hose** | Time: **7 Minutes**
Type: **Strength** | Level: **Beginner**
Goal: **Strength** | Intensity: **40%**

(1) Side Knee Kicks

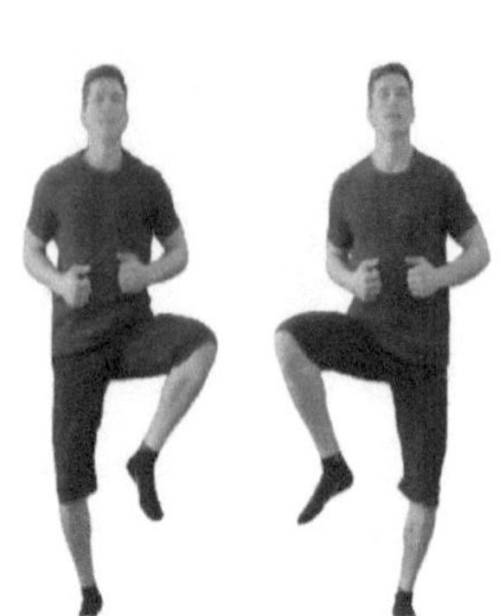

Raise your knee to the side of your body. While lowering the leg in the air raise the other knee, never touching the ground with both feet at the same time.

60 Seconds

(2) Twist Jacks

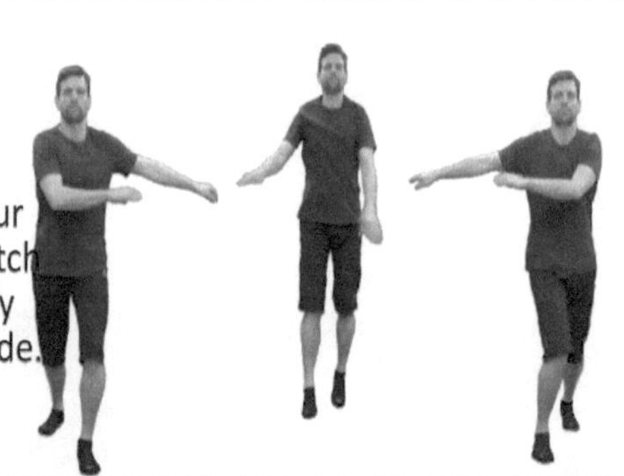

Jump up moving one leg forward and the other backward. Move your arms to the side. Jump up and switch legs in midair, while simultaneously swinging your arms to the other side.

60 Seconds

(3) Side Lunges

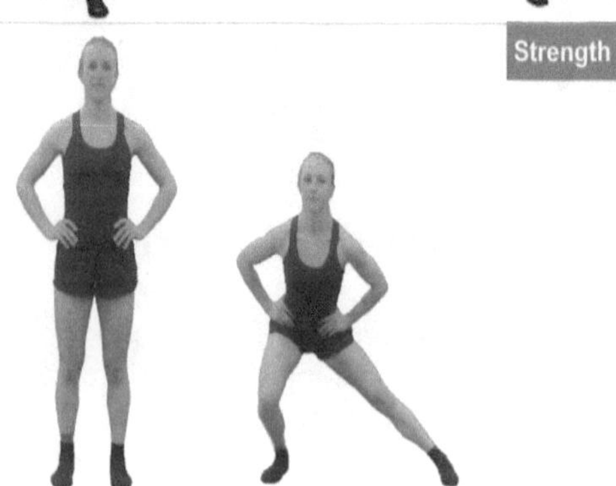

Take a large step to the side and bend your knee no more than 90 degrees. Explode back to the starting position and switch.

10 Reps (per leg)

(4) Leg Extensions

Raise one foot into the air, while keeping your knee at 90 degrees. Stop the lift just before your hips begin to shift. Hold the position briefly and lower your leg to repeat on the other side.

10 Reps (per side)

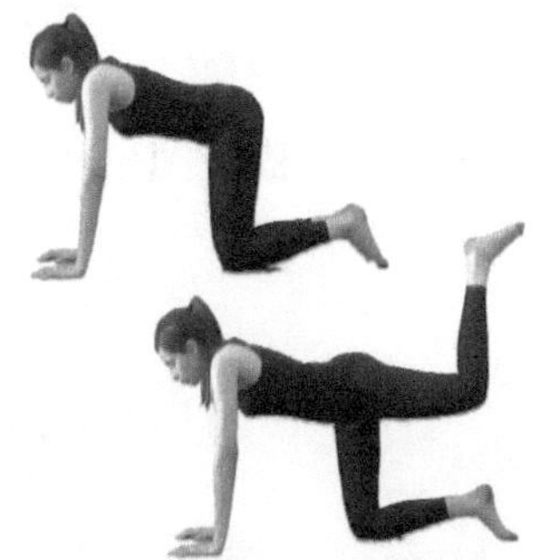

(5) Side Leg Lift

Lay on your side and use your elbow and the hand on the floor to support your body. Point your toes slightly outward at the top to engage your inner glutes.

10 Reps (per side)

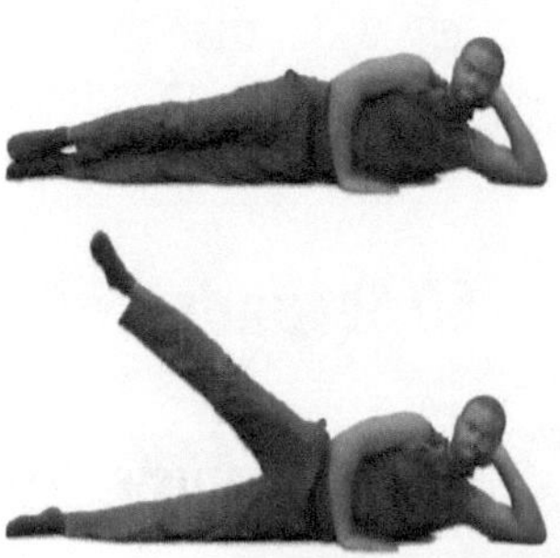

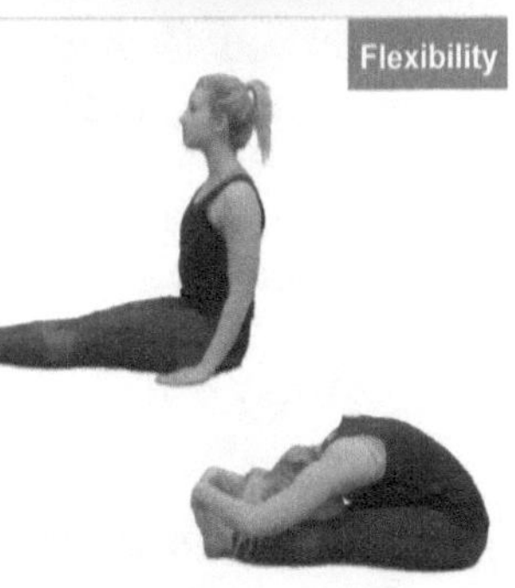

(6) Full Forward Bend Pose

Hinge forward from your hips, pull your shoulders back and relax your neck, while moving closer toward your legs with your pecs. Once you begin to feel the stretch in your legs reach forward with your arms.

2x 30 Seconds

(7) Sage's Pose

Bend your left knee and position your foot flat on the ground on the other side of your leg. Twist your body and move the opposite arm over the bent knee. Push your knee with your elbow to the opposite side.

2x30 Seconds (per side)

Name: **Liberty Push |** Time: **7 Minutes**

Type: **Strength** | Level: **Intermediate**
Goal: **Strength** | Intensity: **60%**

(1)   **Wide Knee Butt kicks**

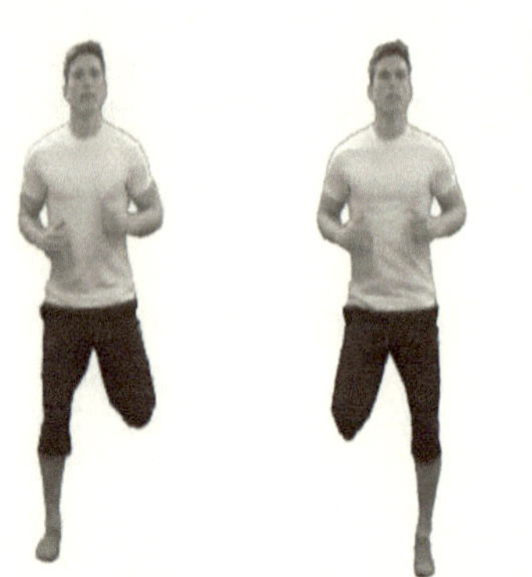

Move in one spot with your legs wider than shoulder-width apart. Lift your heels towards your glutes.

60 Seconds

(2)   **Squat Thrusts**

Kick your leg back to land in a pushup position. Bring your legs forward and stand up to repeat the movement.

20 Reps

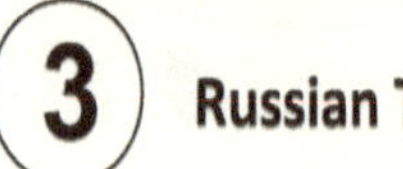

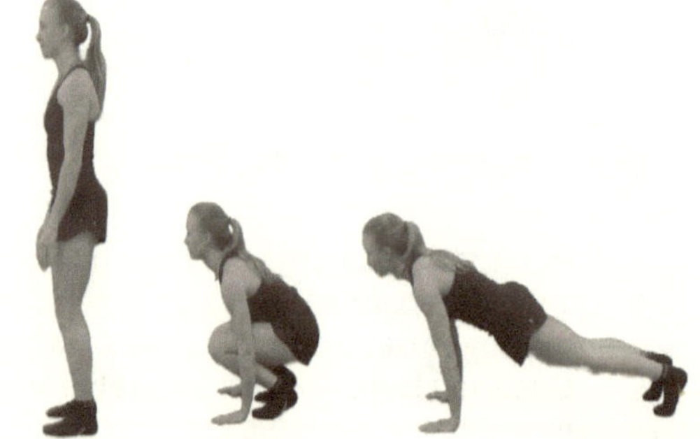

(3)   **Russian Twists**

Twist your body from left to right, moving your elbows past your knees.

60 Seconds

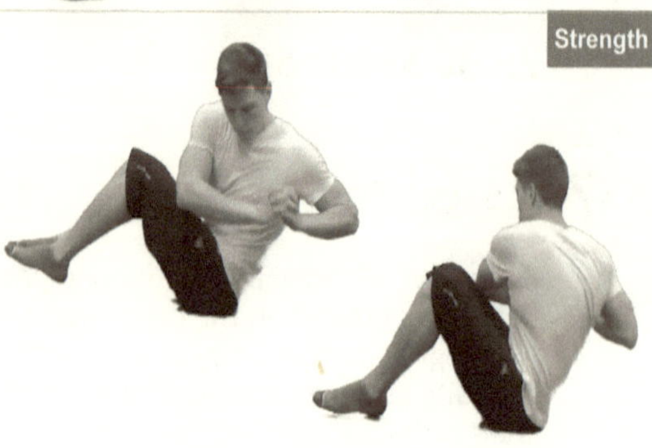

4 S&M Push ups

Lift one leg straight up behind you and lift the opposite arm in front of you. Form a parallel line to the ground with your raised arm and leg.

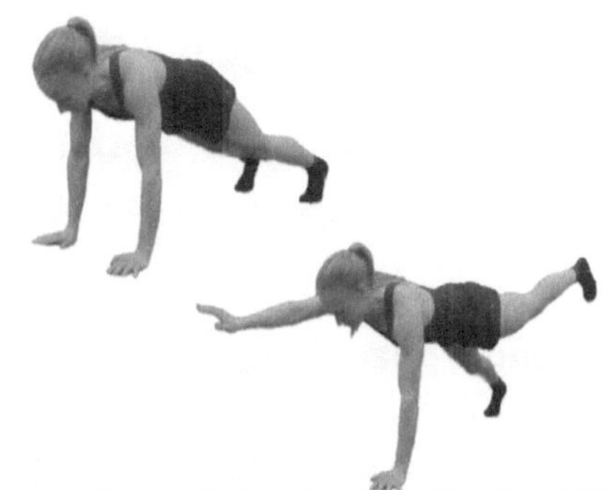

10 Reps (per side)

5 Side Plank Star

Raise your arm and upper leg simultaneously and hold the top position briefly before lowering.

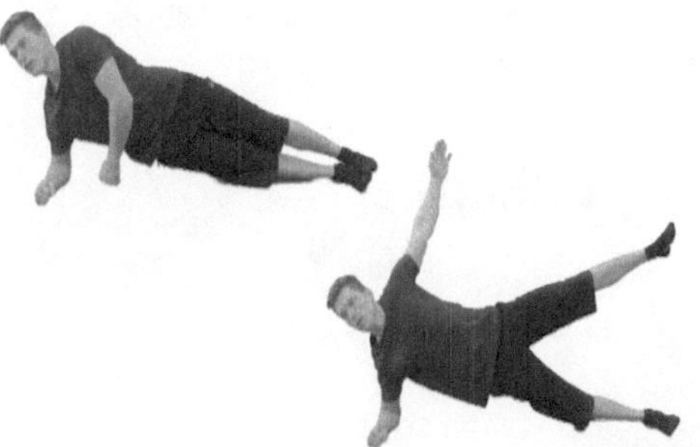

10 Reps (per side)

6 Groin and Back Stretch

Sit on the floor with the soles of your feet together. Interlock your fingers behind your head. Curl downward, moving your elbows in front of your knees.

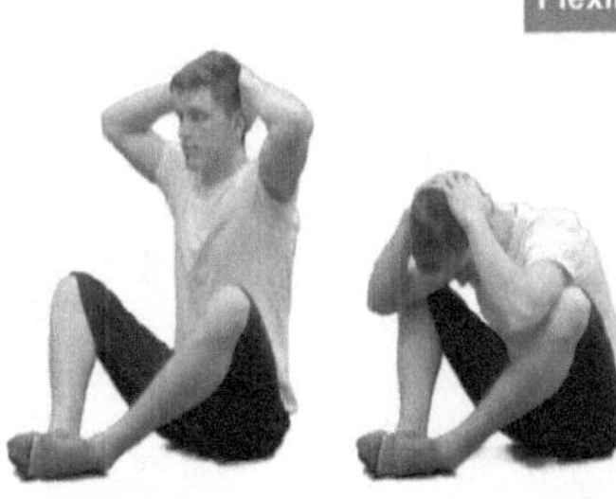

2X30 Seconds

7 Child's Pose

Reach with your arms forward and sit back on your heels. Slowly extend the reach forward with your hands. Lower your pecs closer to the ground as the arms reach farther forward.

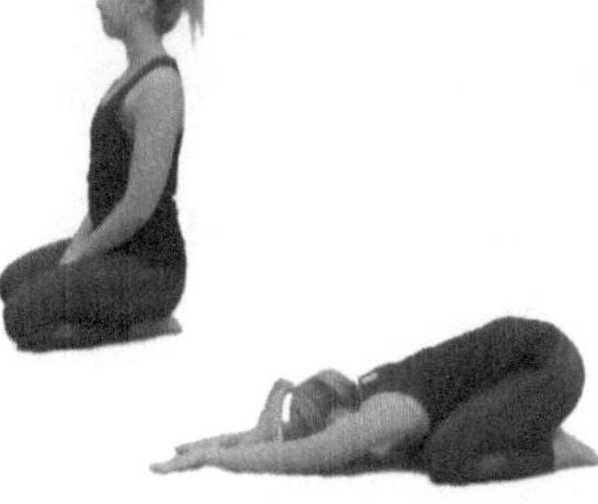

2X30 Seconds

Name: **Rubber Band |** Time: **7 Minutes**

Type: **Cardio, Flexibility |** Level: **Beginner**
Goal: **Endurance, Flexibility |** Intensity: **50%**

1. Jump Knee Tucks

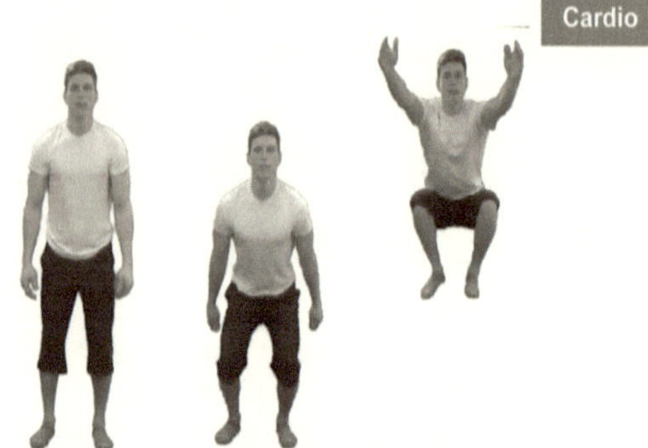

Move down into a squat and explode up tucking your knees into your chest and swinging your arms forward.

15 Reps

2. Squat & Uppercut

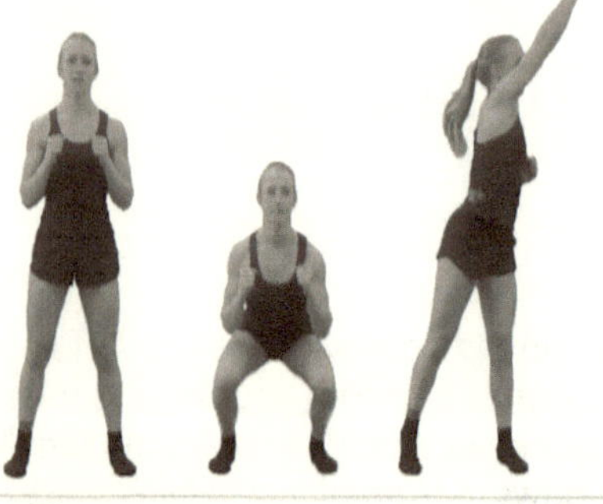

Perform a squat by moving your glutes down until your knees are at a 90 degree angle and explode upward punching to the side.

10 Reps (per side)

3. Plank Jacks

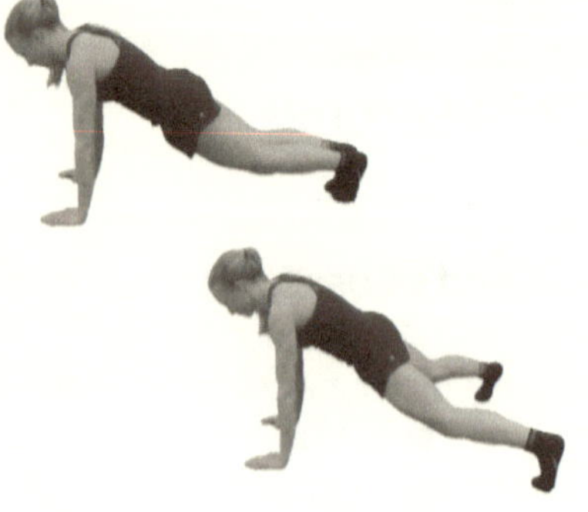

Get into a pushup position. Slightly push off the ground with your legs and spread them apart. Push off the ground again with your legs to return to the starting position.

60 Seconds

4 Step Through's

Get into a push up position.
Move your knee toward the
opposite elbow by lifting you hips
slightly. Return to the starting
position to repeat on the
other side.

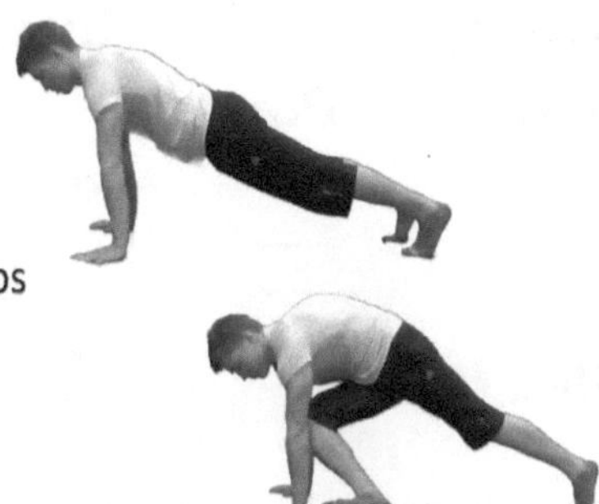

60 Seconds

5 Standing One-legged Ham Stretch

Flexibility

Position one foot in front of the other, bend
your back leg and raise your toes. Lean
forward and keep the front leg straight.

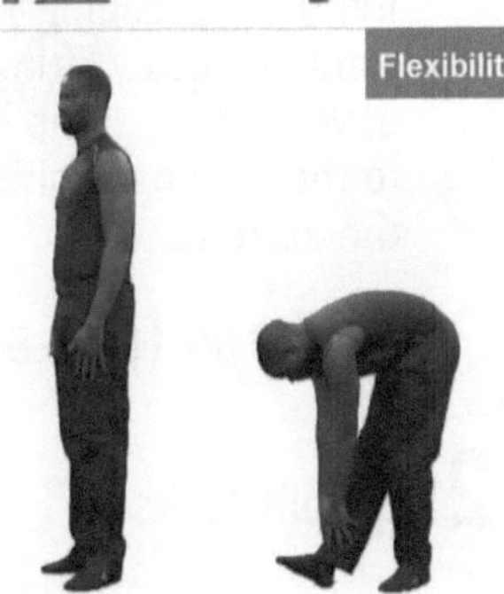

4x15 Seconds

6 Wide-legged Forward Bend II

Lift your hands above your head and hinge
forward from your hips and lower your upper
body toward the floor. Stick your glutes into
the air, while moving your hands behind your
body on the ground.

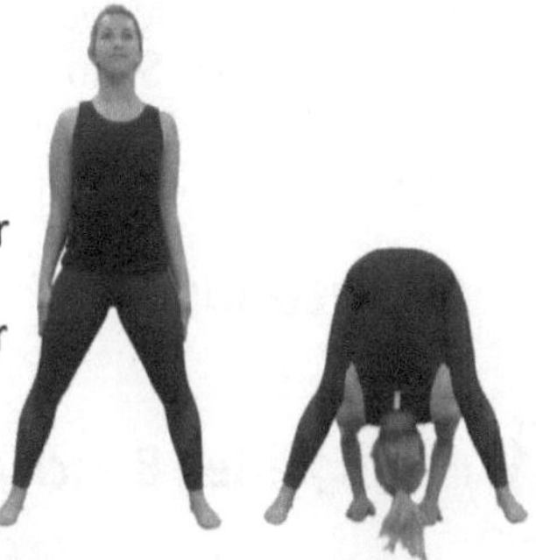

2x30 Seconds

7 Standing Back Bend

Stand upright with your hands
pushing into your lower back.
Move your elbows closer together
and gaze upward.

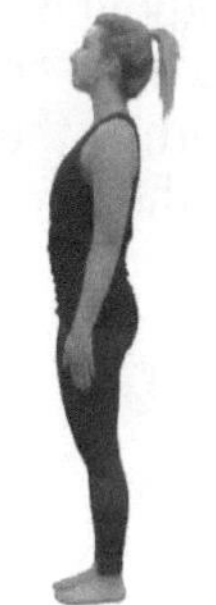

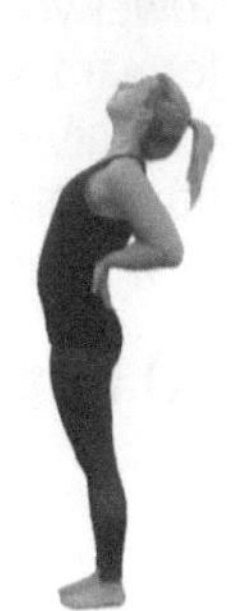

4x15 Seconds

Name: **Leg Greed |** Time: **7 Minutes**
Type: **Strength** | Level: **Intermediate**
Goal: **Strength, Power** | Intensity: **60%**

(1) Fly Jacks

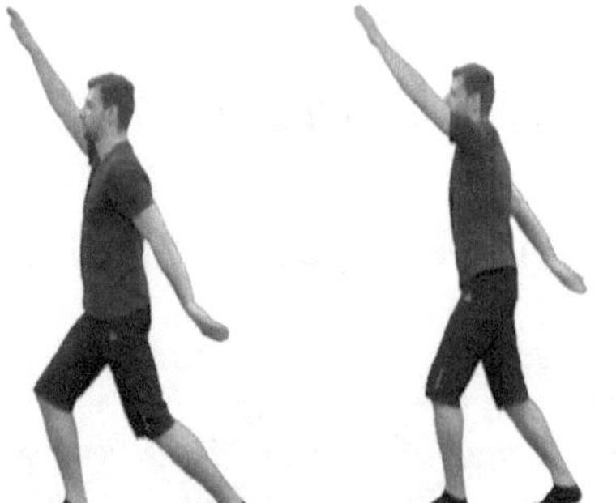

Jump up spreading your legs apart, while simultaneously lifting your arms in front of your chest. Jump back up to return to the starting position and repeat the exercise.

10 Reps (per side)

(2) Split Jacks

Swing one arm forward and the other back. Simultaneously switch the order of your legs and arms in midair.

60 Seconds

(3) Single-leg Bench Get-up

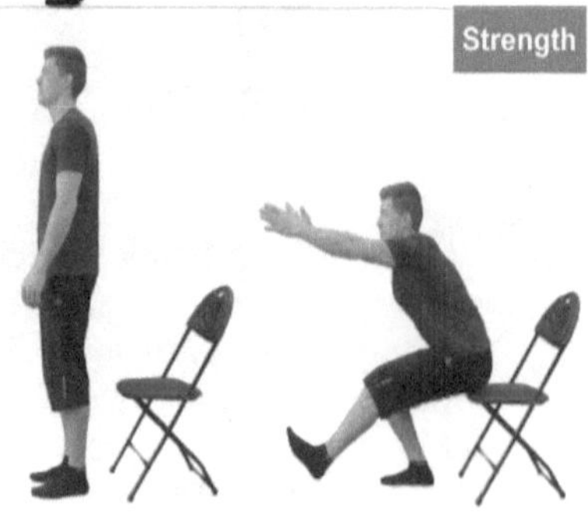

Lower your body without leaning forward. Gently touch the chair with your glutes and return to the starting position. Repeat on the same side with your arms and leg lifted.

10 Reps (per side)

 **Bulgarian Split Squat**

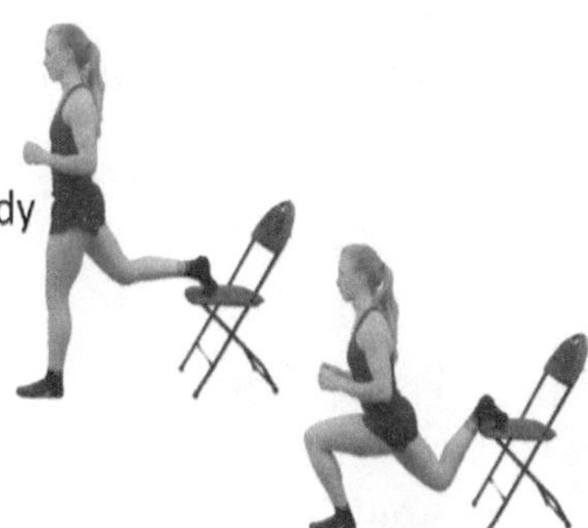

Place one foot on a chair. Lower your body until your knee is at a 90-degree angle. Press onto the floor with your foot to help stabilize your body and to raise your hips back to the starting position.

10 Reps (per side)

 **Chair Jump step-up**

Push your body up with your foot on the chair to jump into the air. Land with your opposite leg on the chair.

30 Reps

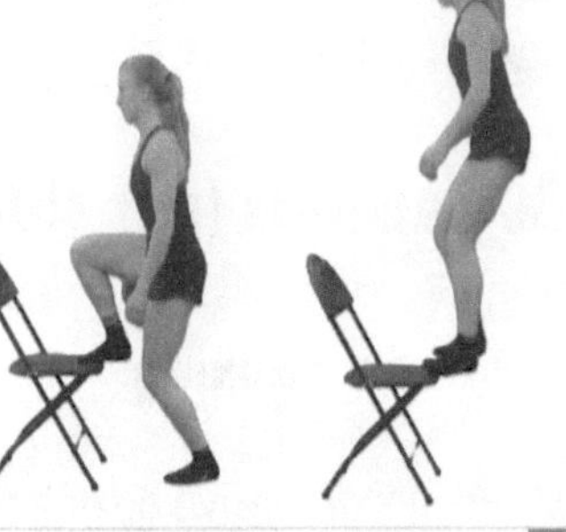

Flexibility

Side Quad Stretch

Lay on your side holding on to the ankle of your upper leg. Press your hip forward and pull the foot of the bent leg toward your lower back without shifting your hips.

30 Seconds (per side)

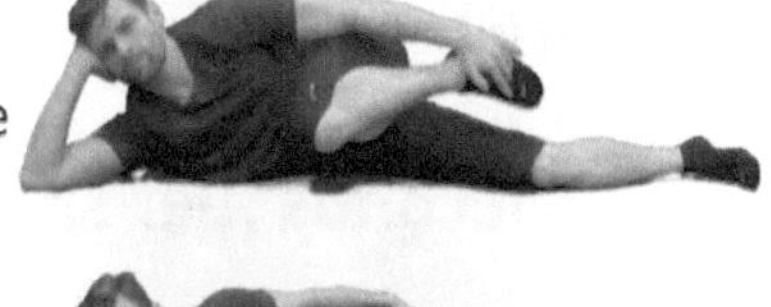

 **Supine One-legged Stretch**

Straighten the bent leg and reach toward your calf. Pull your leg back using the weight of your body. Keep both legs straight while lowering your upper-body back toward the ground.

30 Seconds (per side)

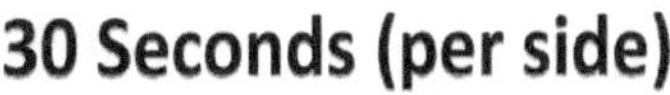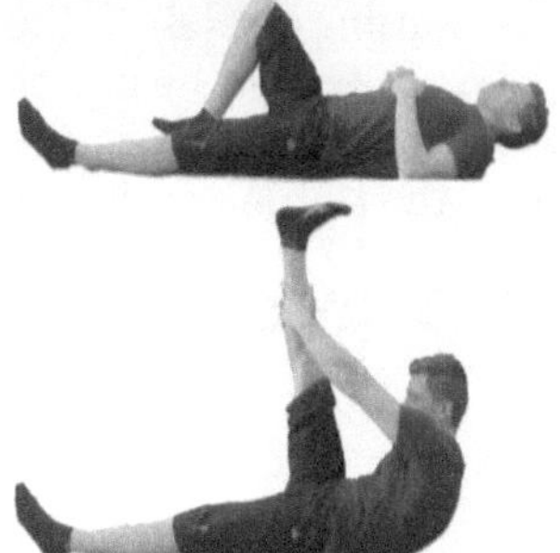

Name: **Ring Side |** Time: **7 Minutes**

Type: **Strength** | Level: **Beginner**
Goal: **Strength** | Intensity: **40%**

1. Front Kicks

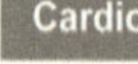

Kick with the leg in front by lifting your knee into the air and flicking the leg forward. Return to the starting position and repeat with the same foot.

30 Seconds (per side)

2. Shadow Boxing

Stand in a defensive boxing position and punch forward interchangably with each arm rotating your body slightly.

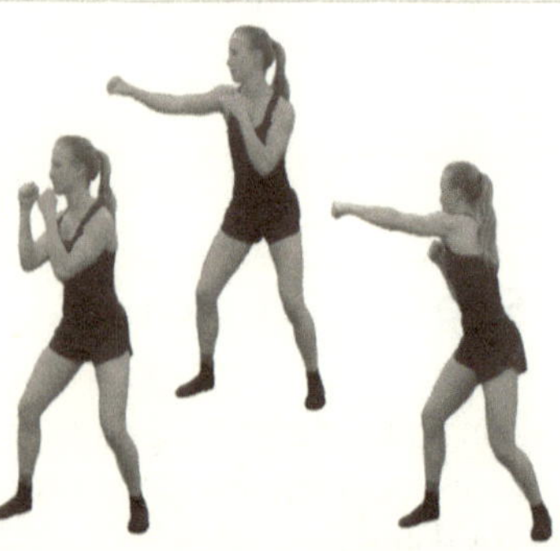

30 Seconds (per side)

3. Chair Dip with Leg Lift

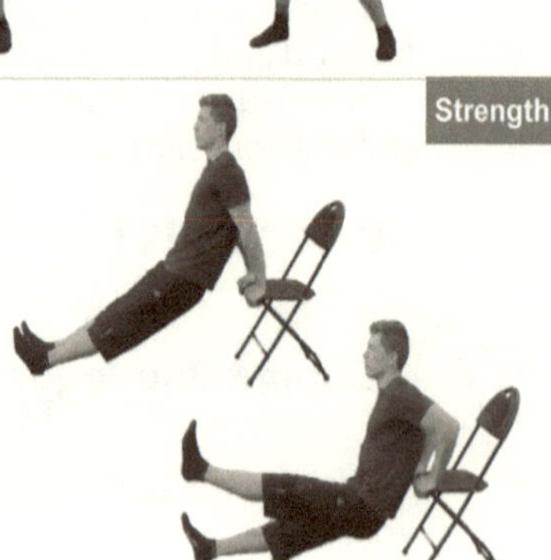

Lower your glutes toward the ground while raising one leg off the ground. Hold the position at the bottom briefly and lower your leg as you raise your body back to the starting position.

5 Reps (per side)

(4) Single-leg Hip Raises

Place the heels of your feet on an elevated suraface. Raise your hips into the air and extend one leg straight into the air. Hold the position at the top for a second and repeat on the same side.

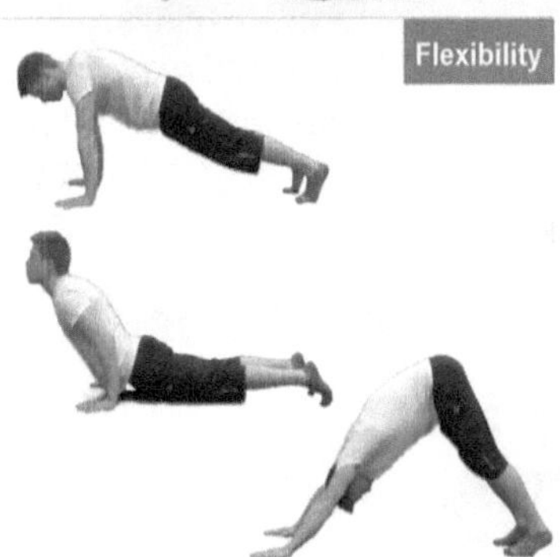

5 Reps (per side)

(5) Modified Diamond Pushup

Get into a pushup position with your knees on the ground and your index fingers and thumbs touching. Lower your body toward the ground and push yourself up forcefully, keeping your elbows bent at the top position.

10 Reps

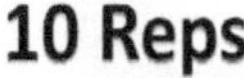

(6) Downward-Facing Dog

Flexibility

Lift your hips into the air, extending your arms and legs to create an inverted V shape with your body. Move your pecs toward your legs, lower your body slowly to the starting position.

10 Reps

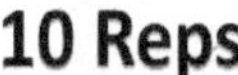

(7) Kneeling Twist

Rotate your torso and reach with your arm straight up as high as possible, leaving the other arm on the ground. Pull your shoulders back and open your pecs.

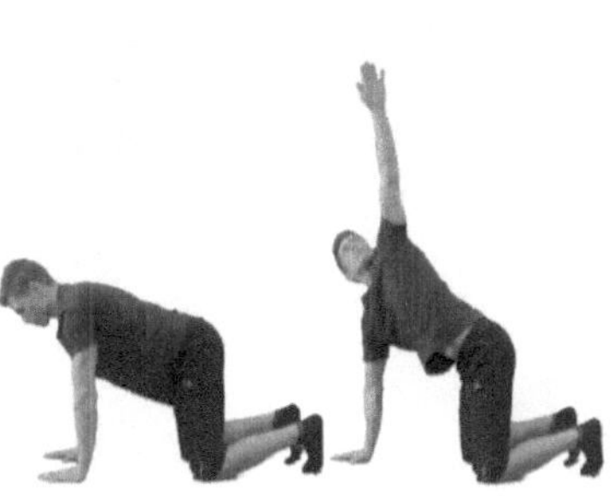

5 Reps (per side)

Name: **Flying Low |** Time: **7 Minutes**

Type: **Flexibility** | Level: **Beginner**
Goal: **Flexibility, Balance** | Intensity: **30%**

(1) **Arm Circles**

Flexibility

Start by making small circles with your arms and slowly progress into making the circles bigger. Repeat going forward or switch to backward circles.

60 Seconds

(2) **Forward Leg Swings**

Perform a backward lunge and stop half way. Swing your back leg forward and reach toward the front foot with with your opposite arm.

2x10 Reps

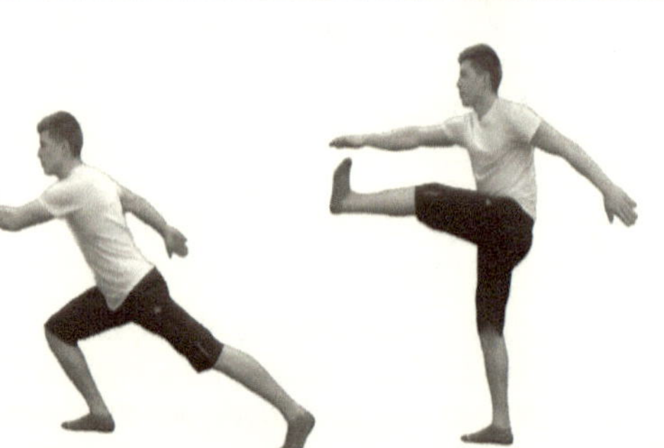

(3) **Step Forwards**

Start in a pushup position, slowly step forward with both legs and raise your hips while reaching toward your feet. Continue to lean forward, while stepping forward.

10 Reps

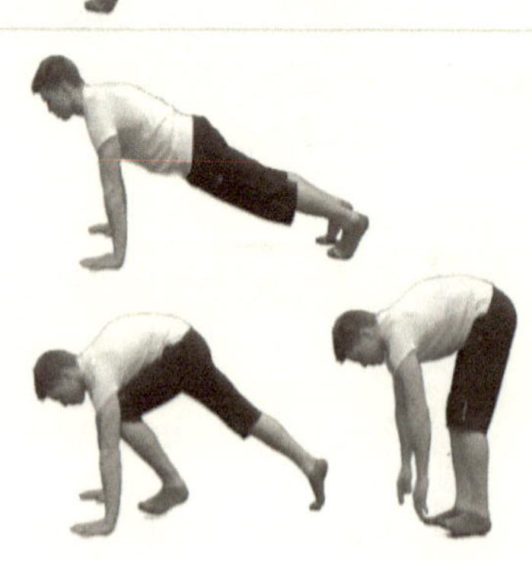

④ Wild Thing (Variation)

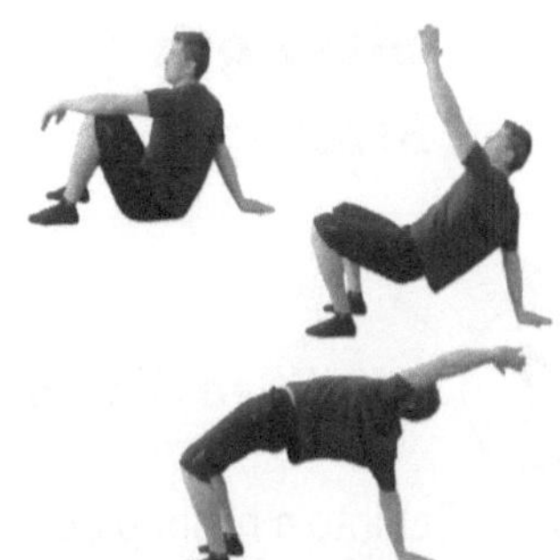

Postion one arm underneath your shoulders. Raise your hips as high as possible, extending the other arm beside your ear and past your head. Briefly hold and return to the starting position to repeat on the other side.

5 Reps (per side)

⑤ Bent-over Reach to the Sky

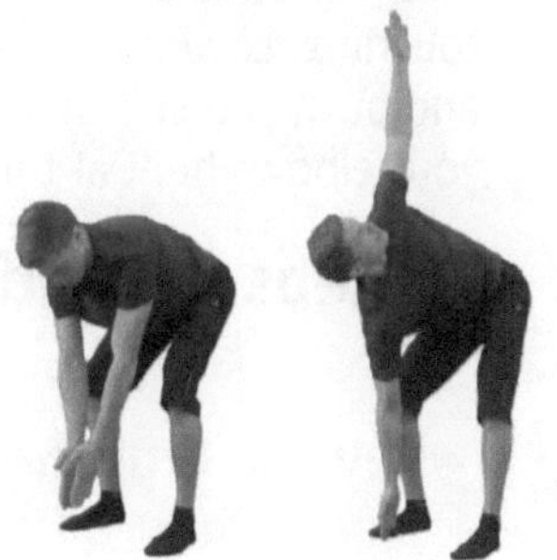

Rotate your torso and reach with your arm as high as possible, creating a vertical line with your arms. Pause at the top and move back to the starting position to repeat on the other side.

60 Seconds

⑥ Standing One-legged Stretch

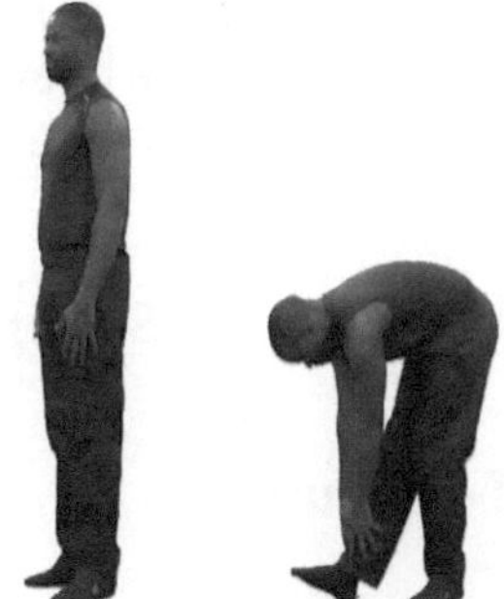

Position one foot in front of the other, bend your back leg slightly and raise the toes of your front foot. Lean forward and keep the front leg straight.

4x15 Seconds

⑦ Standing Soleus Stretch

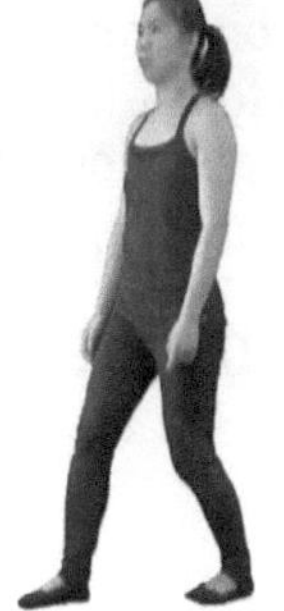

Stand upright and take a small step backward. Lean forward from your knees and keep your feet flat on the ground.

30 Seconds (per side)

Name: **Ground Digger |** Time: **7 Minutes**

Type: **Strength** | Level: **Beginner**
Goal: **Strength** | Intensity: **40%**

1　Modified Diamond Pushup

Get into a pushup position with your knees on the ground and your index fingers and thumbs touching. Lower your body toward the ground and push yourself up forcefully, keeping your elbows bent at the top position.

10 Reps (per side)

2　Reverse Crunches

Contract your abs and then curl your knees toward your pecs keeping your knees at 90 degrees. Pause briefly and slowly lower your legs to the starting position.

10 Reps (per side)

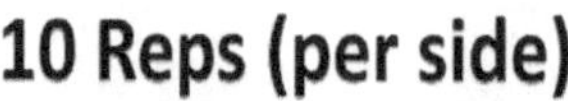

3　T-Pushups

Push up forcefully and twist your body. Extend one arm up until both arms are vertical to the floor. Once your arms are straight, move back into the starting position and repeat on the other side.

10 Reps (per side)

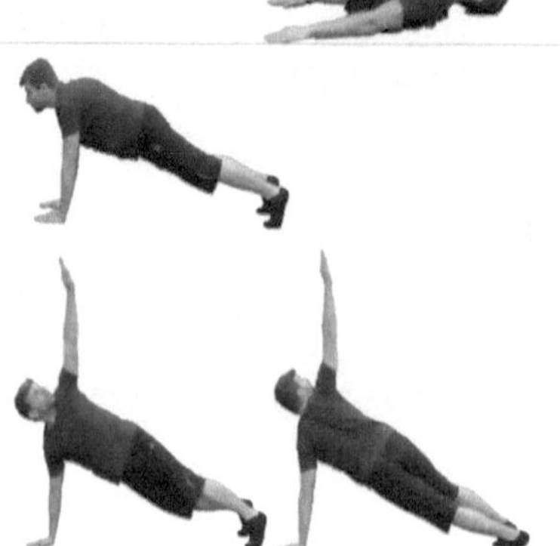

4 Knee-Ins & Twists

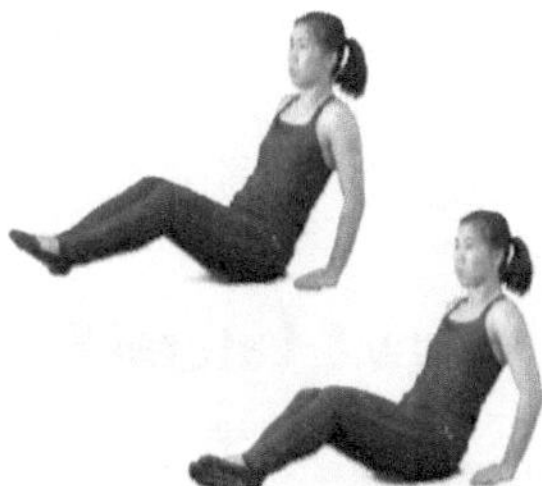

Twist your knees from side to side without touching the ground with your feet. Rotate your lower body, while moving your knees to the other side.

60 Seconds

5 Modified Wide Pushup

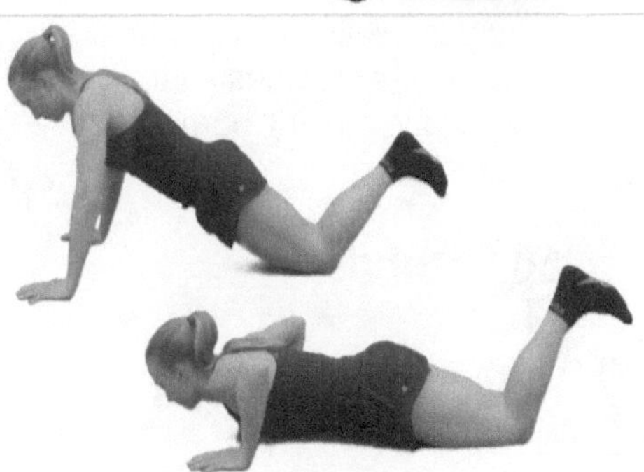

Get into a Pushup position with your arms wider than shoulder-width apart and the weight of your lower body resting on your knees.

60 Seconds

6 Crossed-Arm Crunches

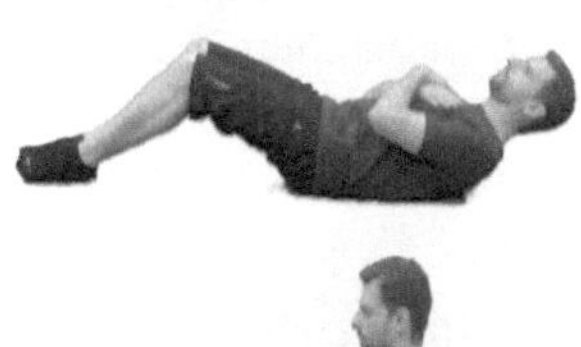

Raise your body until it is in a sitting position at a 45-degree angle to the floor, pause for a second and lower your body to the starting position.

60 Seconds

7 Plank arm raises

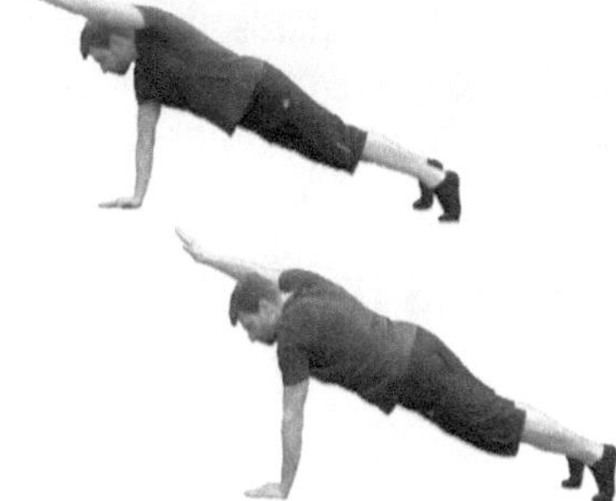

Get into a push up position and lift one arm straight beside your ear. Hold briefly and switch sides.

60 Seconds

Name: **Last Stance** | Time: **7 Minutes**

Type: **Cardio** | Level: **Beginner**
Goal: **Endurance** | Intensity: **40%**

(1) Row & Lateral Steps

Cross one leg behind the other leg, while pulling your shoulders back. Open your chest while moving both elbows back.

60 Seconds

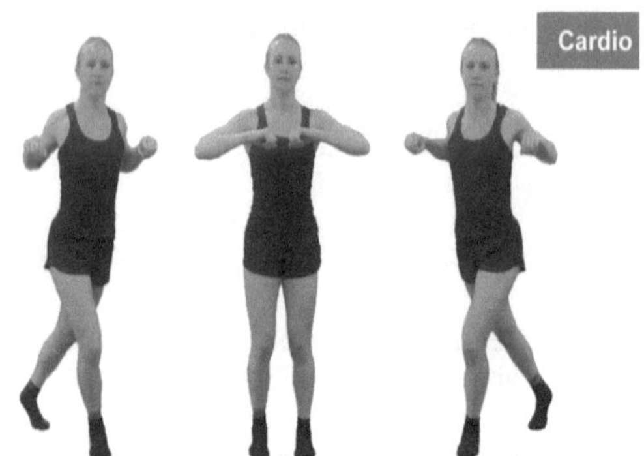

(2) Wide Knee Butt kicks

Move in one spot with your legs wider than shoulder-width apart. Lift your heels towards your glutes.

60 Seconds

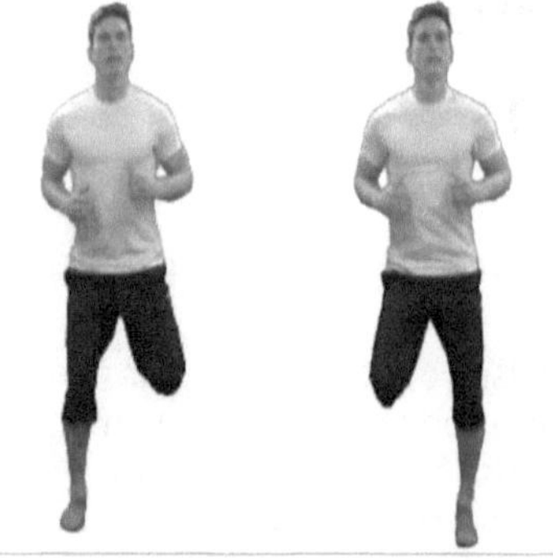

(3) Hip Circles

Raise one knee to the side of your body until the quads are parallel to the floor. Reverse the movement and repeat on the other side.

10 Reps (per side)

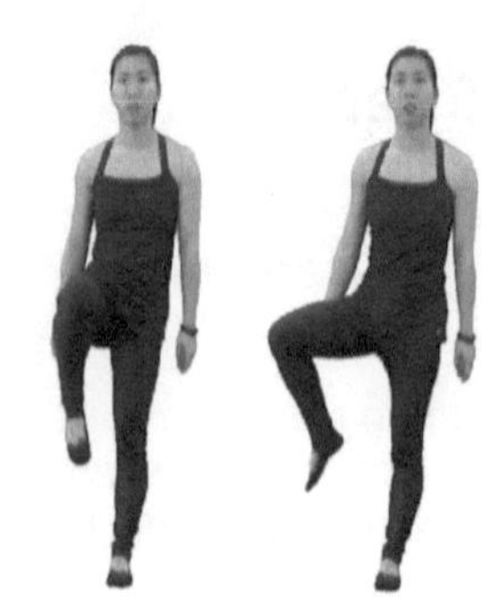

Pushup with Knee Lift

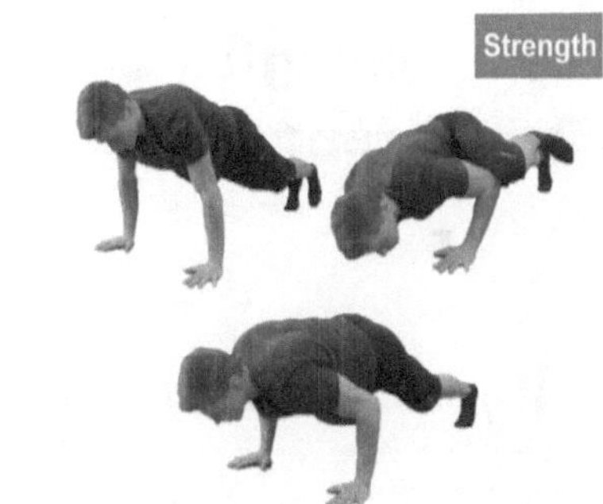

Lower your pecs to perform a pushup and simultaneously bring your knee toward your elbow on the same side. Alternate sides after each pushup.

10 Reps (per side)

Hip Raises

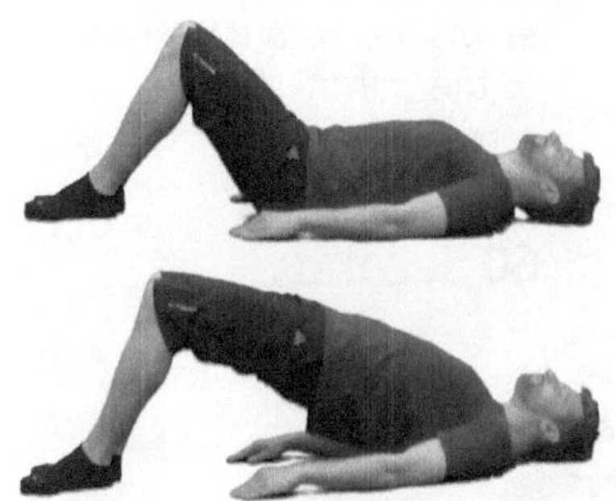

Lift your glutes and clench your core to create a straight line from your pecs to your knees. Hold the top position briefly and move back down to repeat.

60 Seconds

Side Neck Push

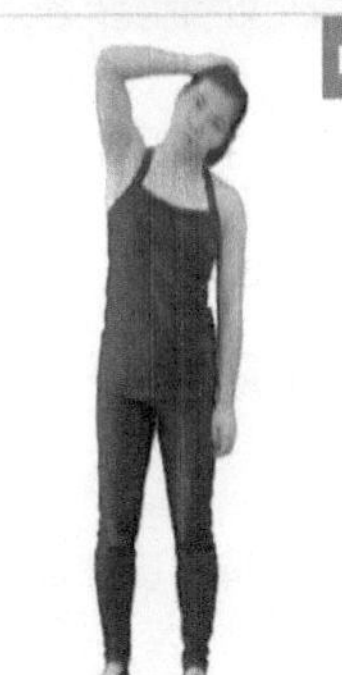

Stand upright placing one hand on the side of your head. Gently push your ear toward your shoulder. Keep the rest of your body relaxed.

2x15 Seconds (per side)

Tree Pose

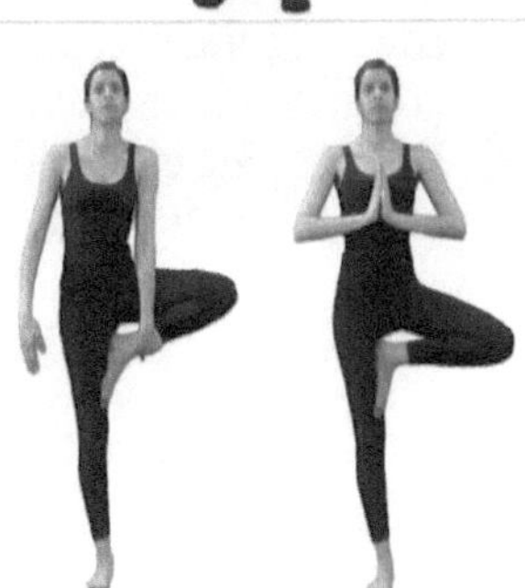

Keep the foot anchored within your inner thigh. Place the palms of your hands together and gaze forward at a still point.

30 Seconds (per side)

Name: **Flame Mix |** Time: **7 Minutes**

Type: **Strength |** Level: **Intermediate**
Goal: **Strength |** Intensity: **60%**

① Mountain Climbers

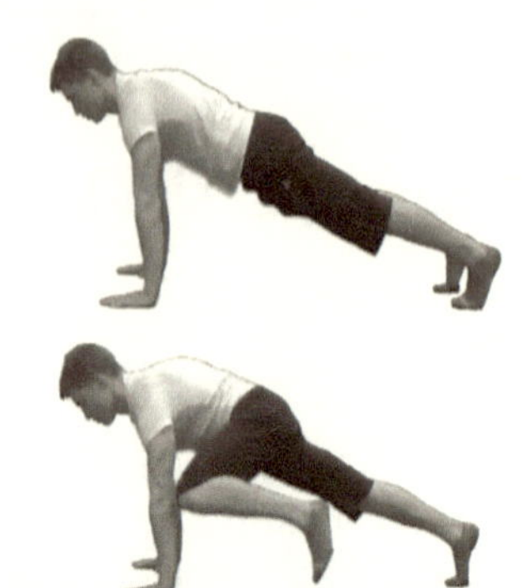

Lift your knee toward your elbow and return your foot to the starting position to repeat with your other leg.

60 Seconds

② Squat Thrusts

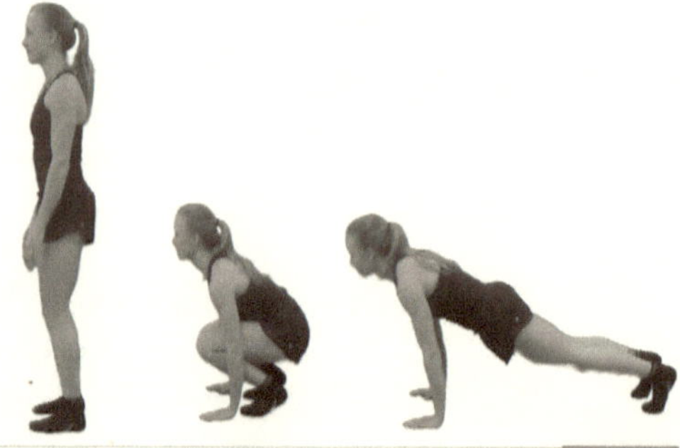

Kick your leg back to land in a pushup position. Bring your legs forward and stand up to repeat the movement.

20 Reps

③ Chair dip with leg lift

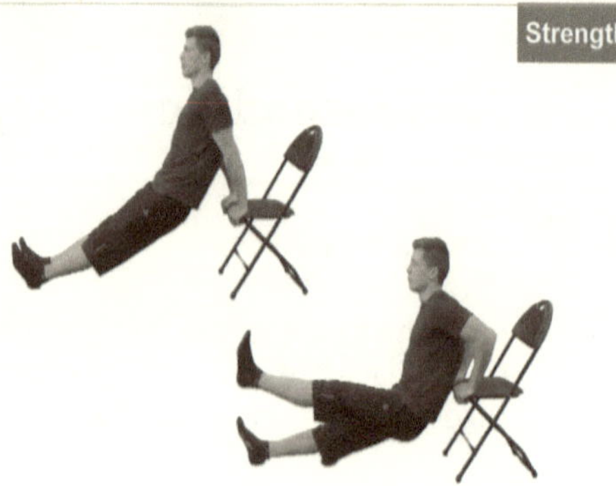

Lower your glutes towards the ground and raise one leg. Keep the leg elevated, while lowering and raising your hips.

10 Reps (per side)

(4) Single-leg Bench Get-up

Lower your body without leaning forward. Gently touch the chair with your glutes and return to the starting position. Repeat on the same side with your arms and leg lifted.

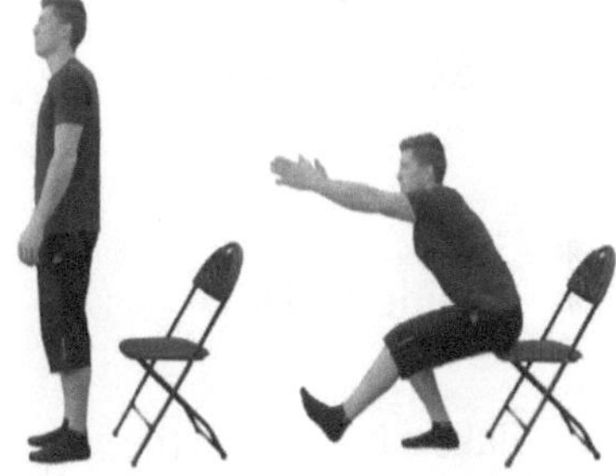

10 Reps (per side)

(5) Single-leg Hip Raises

Place the heels of your feet on an elevated suraface. Raise your hips into the air and extend one leg straight into the air. Hold the position at the top for a second and repeat on the same side.

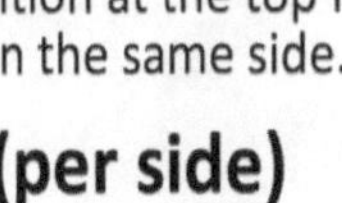

10 Reps (per side)

(6) Seated Hip Stretch

Place the ankle of one foot on top of the quad of the other foot. Press the knee down to open your hips.

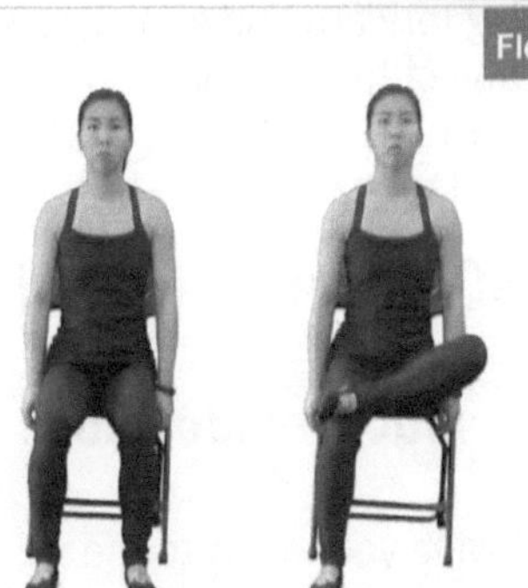

2x15 Seconds (per side)

(7) Seated Side Bend

Reach over your head with one arm and reach toward the opposite side. Reach to the side as far as possible without lifting your glutes off the chair.

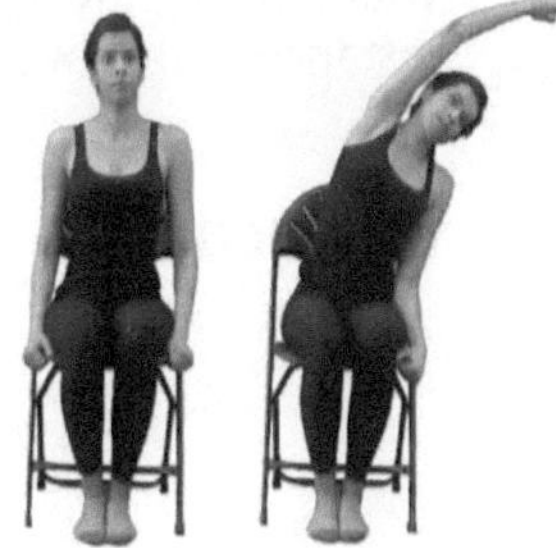

2x15 Seconds (per side)

Name: **Twister |** Time: **7 Minutes**
Type: **Strength** | Level: **Beginner**
Goal: **Strength** | Intensity: **40%**

1 Side Jacks

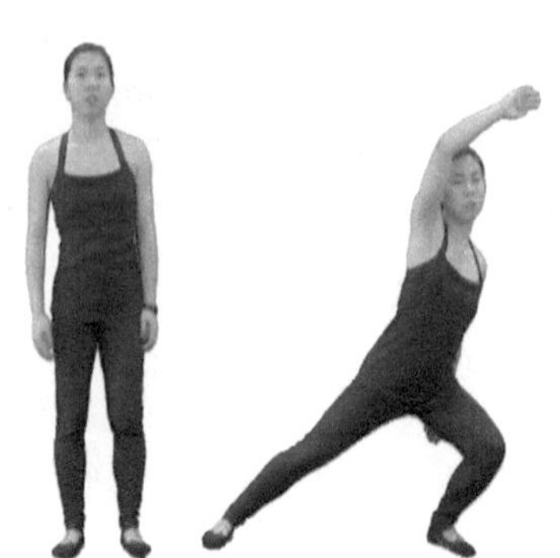

Take a big step to the side, while reaching over your head with your arm.

60 Seconds

2 Low Kick

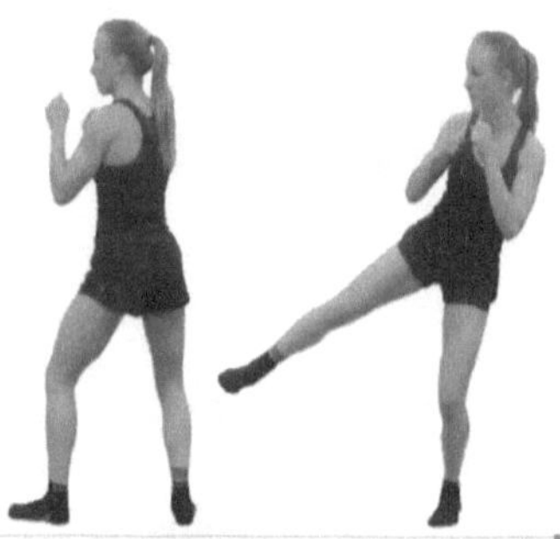

Turn your body, extending your back leg forward and aiming toward an object that is at knee height. Pull your leg back to the starting position and repeat on the same side.

30 Seconds (per side)

3 Side-to-Side Chops

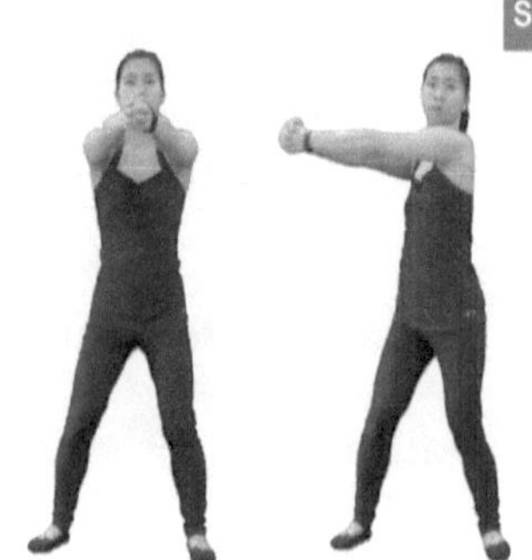

Swing your arms to the side, keeping your hands at the same height. Rotate your hips slightly to increase the distance of the swing.

60 Seconds

4 Air Bike Crunches

Lift both legs off the ground and begin to paddle as if you were riding a bike.

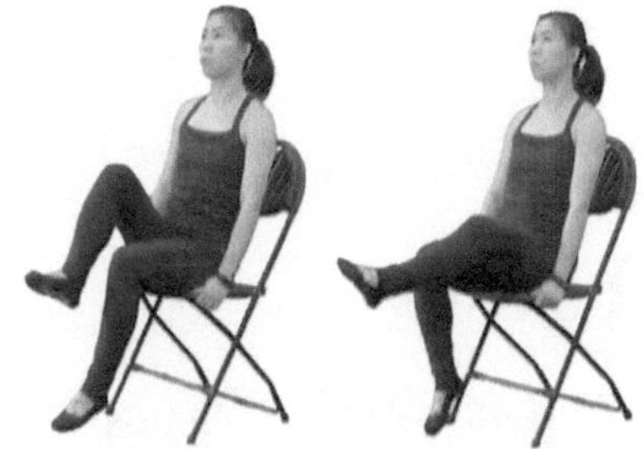

60 Seconds

5 Chair Pose

Lower into a squat position while simultaneously raising your arms. Move your arms straight over your head in line with your ears and stay in a squat position.

2x30 Seconds

6 Good Mornings

Flexibility

Hinge forward from the hips and bend your knees slightly. Contract your core as you slowly move down and up with your upper body. Hold the position briefly and move back to the starting position.

2x30 Seconds

7 Lotus Pose

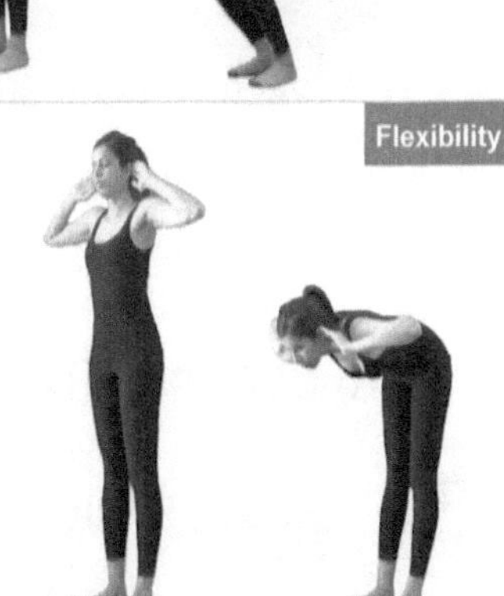

Position your legs on top of each other. Place the back of your hands on top of your knees and breathe deeply.

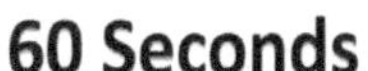

60 Seconds

Name: **Lifter |** Time: **7 Minutes**

Type: **Flexibility, Strength** | Level: **Beginner**
Goal: **Flexibility. Strength** | Intensity: **40%**

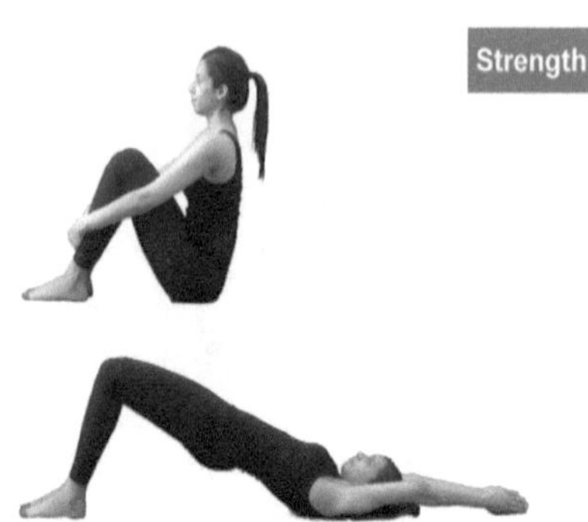

(1) Bridges

Lay down on the floor, keeping your knees bent and raise your arms over your head. Raise your hips into the air until your body forms a straight line from the knees to the shoulders.

20 Reps

(2) Side Plank

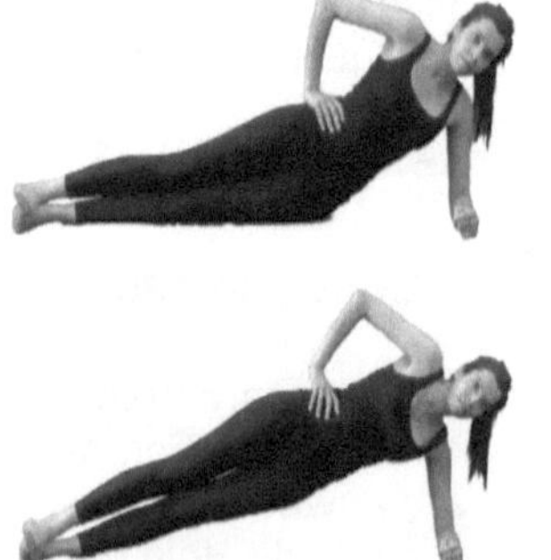

Lift your hips off the ground and form a straight line from your feet to your head. Clench your abs and oblique's briefly at the top position.

30 Seconds (per side)

(3) Knee to Elbows

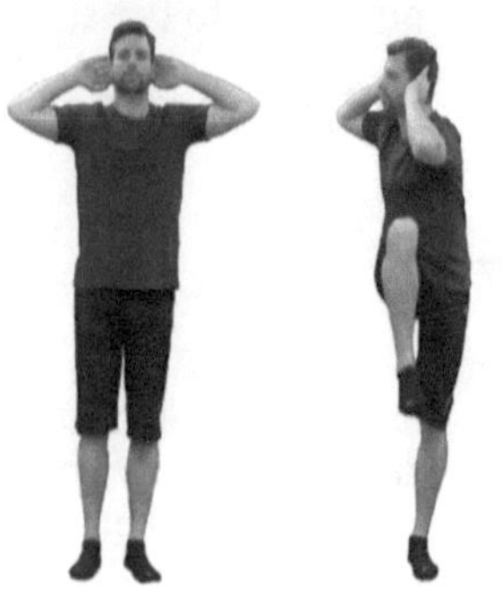

Twist your body and move your elbow toward the opposite knee. Lift your knee off the ground as high as possible, without rotating your pelvis. Return to the starting position to repeat on the other side.

60 Seconds

(4) Reverse Table Top

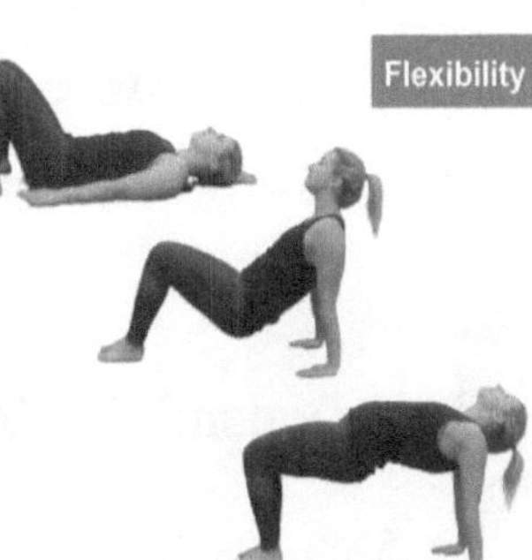

Move your hands underneath your shoulders and lift your upper body off the ground. Raise your hips to create a straight line from your shoulders to your knees. Extend your arms and gaze upward.

4x15 Seconds

(5) Upper back-leg grab

Sit on the floor with your knees slightly bent. Move your chest toward your knees and wrap your arms around your legs.

2x30 Seconds

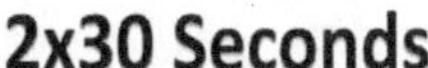

(6) Seated Butterfly

Pull the feet closer toward your groin and sit tall. To stretch the groin, push your legs down using your elbows.

2x30 Seconds

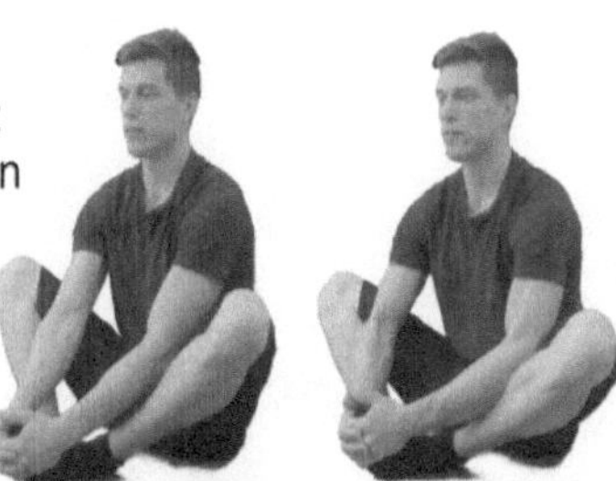

(7) Seated Calf Stretch

Extend one foot in front and tuck the other foot into your groin. Reach toward the toes and pull them back.

30 Seconds (per side)

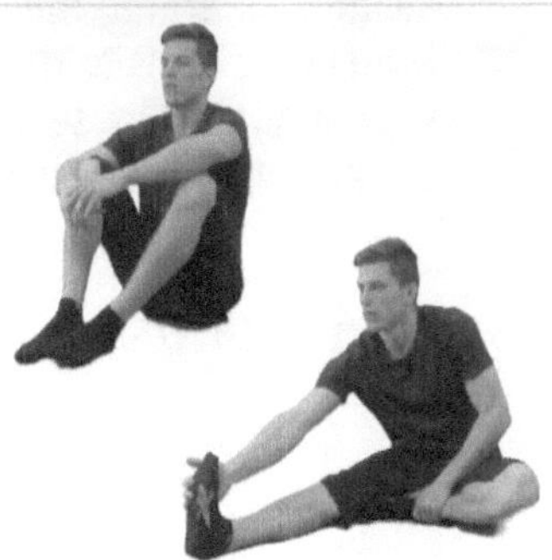

Name: **Hurricane |** Time: **7 Minutes**
Type: **Flexibility, Strength** | Level: **Beginner**
Goal: **Flexibility Strength** | Intensity: **40%**

(1) **Dynamic Pec Stretch**

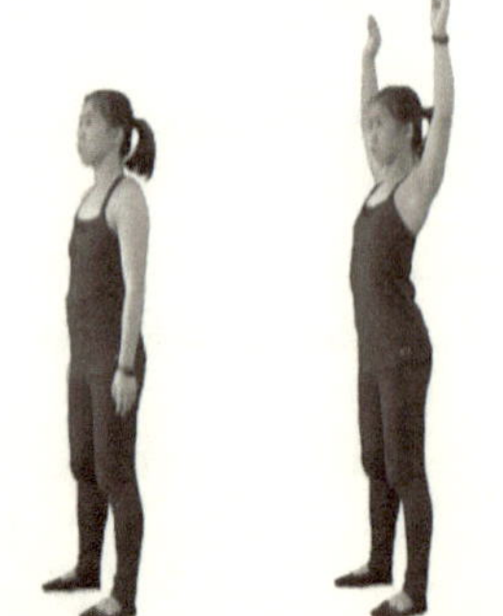

Swing your arms back as far as possible behind your back, positioning them parallel to the ground. Move your arms back together to repeat.

60 Seconds

(2) **Dynamic Back Stretch**

Swing your arms slightly back to stretch your lats. Try to swing your arms behind your head at the top position.

60 Seconds

(3) **Upper-body Rotations**

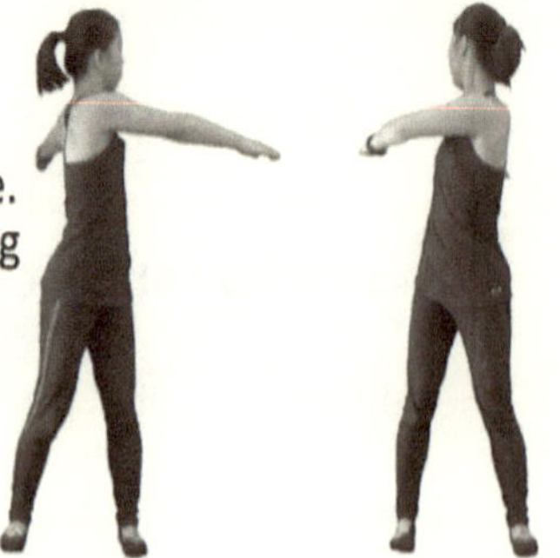

Swing your arm to the side rotating your core. Swing your arms to the opposite side, keeping your shoulders loose. Keep your feet flat on the ground during the entire movement.

60 Seconds

④ Leg Extensions

Raise one foot into the air, while keeping your knee at 90 degrees. Stop the lift just before your hips begin to shift. Hold the position briefly and lower your leg to repeat on the other side.

10 Reps (per side)

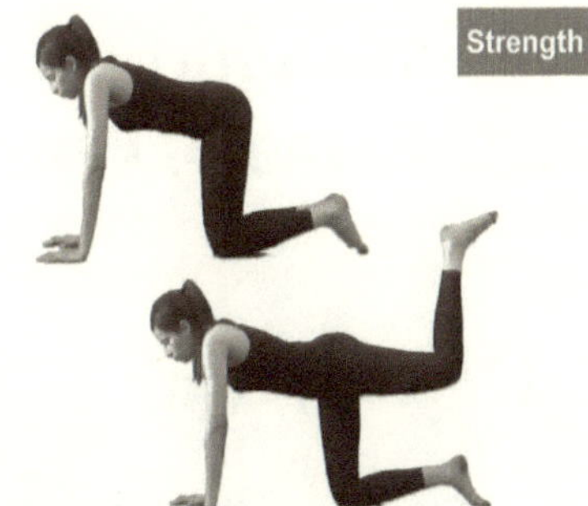

⑤ Inchworm

Walk with your hands forward until you are in a pushup position. Reverse the entire motion to get back to the starting position.

10 Reps

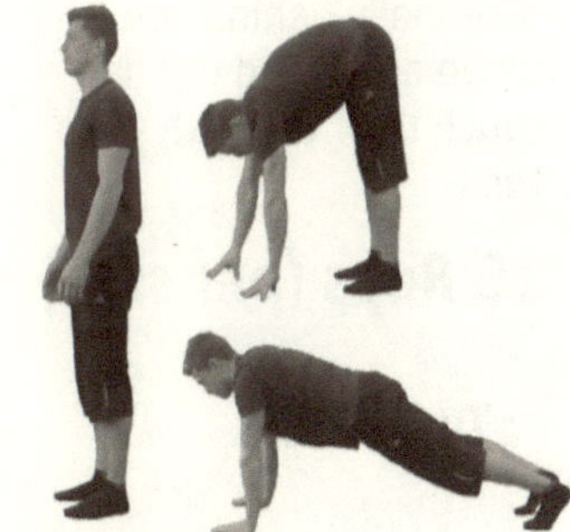

⑥ Bicycles

Lay on your back and lift both feet off the ground. Pull your left knee toward your chest and move it back to the starting position while simultaniously pulling the other knee toward your chest.

60 Seconds

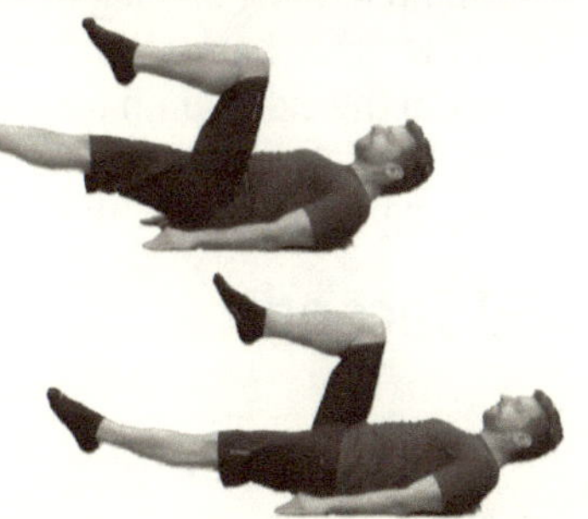

⑦ Clam Shells

Lie on your side and lift your upper knee off the ground and keep both heels together. Stop your knee lift just before your body begins to shift its weight backward.

10 Reps (per side)

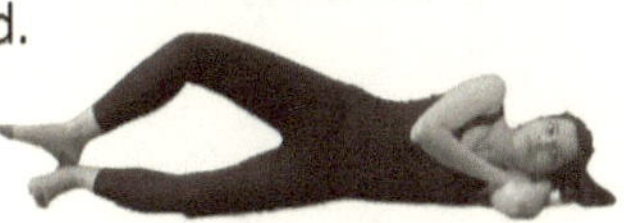

Name: **Home Opener |** Time: **7 Minutes**
Type: **Strength |** Level: **Intermediate**
Goal: **Strength, Power |** Intensity: **70%**

1 Curtsy Squat

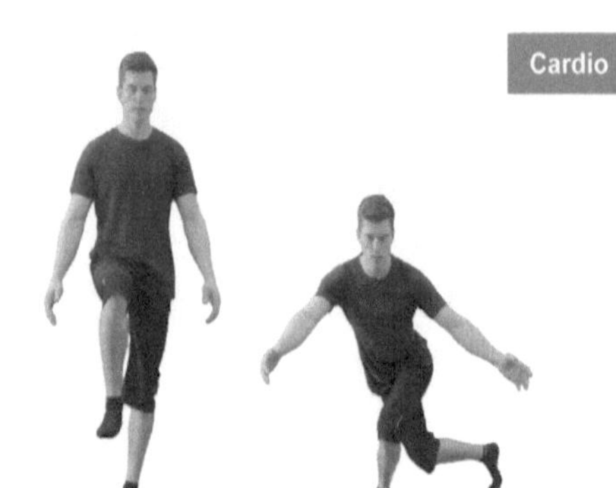

Cross your lifted leg diagonally behind you, lunge down and briefly touch the floor with you toes.

10 Reps (per side)

2 Twist Jacks

Jump up moving one leg forward and the other backward. Move your arms to the side. Jump up and switch legs in midair, while simultaneously swinging your arms to the other side

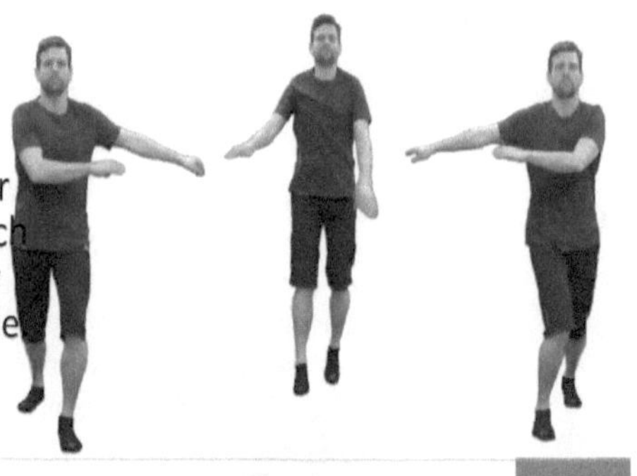

60 Seconds

3 Plank to Pushup

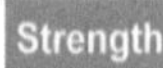

Start in a plank position with the forearms flat on the ground. Lift your arms off the ground to get into a pushup position and reverse the movement to move back into a plank to repeat the exercise.

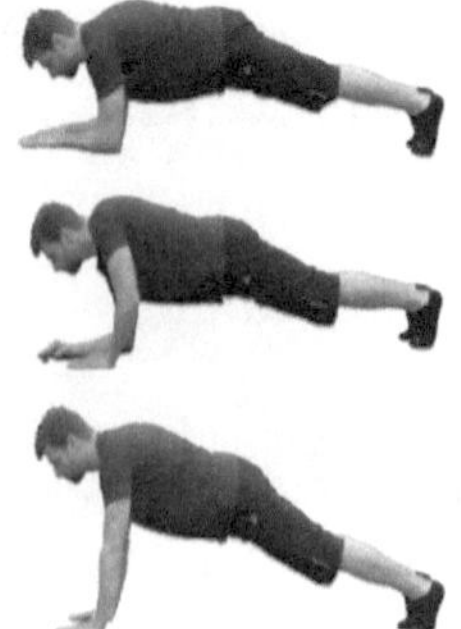

60 Seconds

(4) Butt-ups

Extend your legs straight into the air, using your arms to push your legs upward. Slowly lower your legs back to the starting position without touching the ground to repeat.

10 Reps

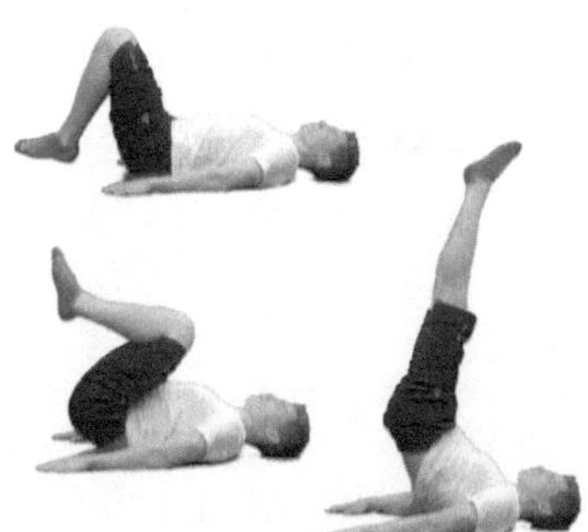

(5) Side Plank with Reach Under

Extend your arm straight up, following your hand with your gaze. Rotate your hips slightly to reach under and behind your body. Move your arm straight up again and repeat on the same side.

10 Reps (per side)

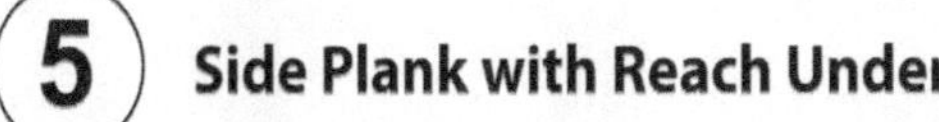

Flexibility

(6) Head-down Hero Pose

Slowly lean forward with your upper-body and place your hands over your head. Walk your hands forward as your upper-body is moving closer to the floor. Move your head between your knees, stretching your lats.

2x30 Seconds

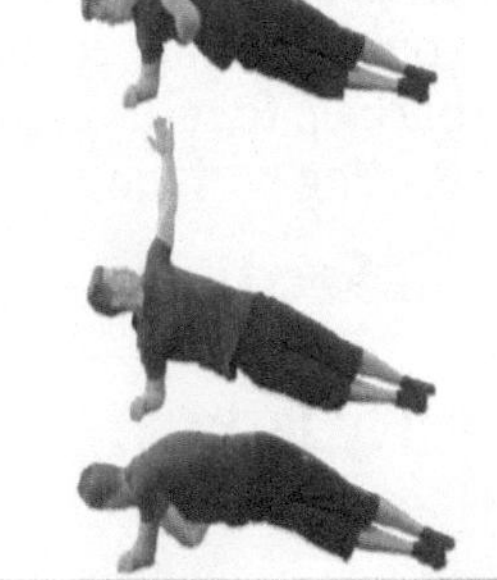

(7) Reclining Knee-Hug Stretch

Lift your knees off the ground and wrap your arms around your knees. Gently pull your knees closer toward your pecs.

2x30 Seconds

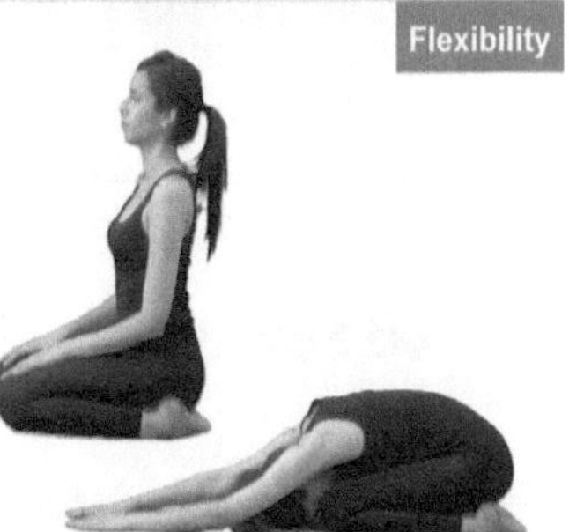
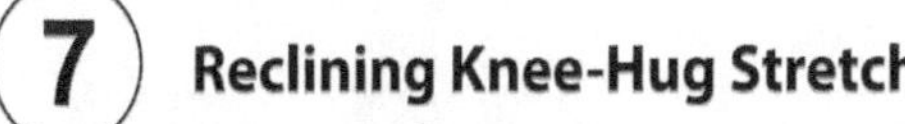
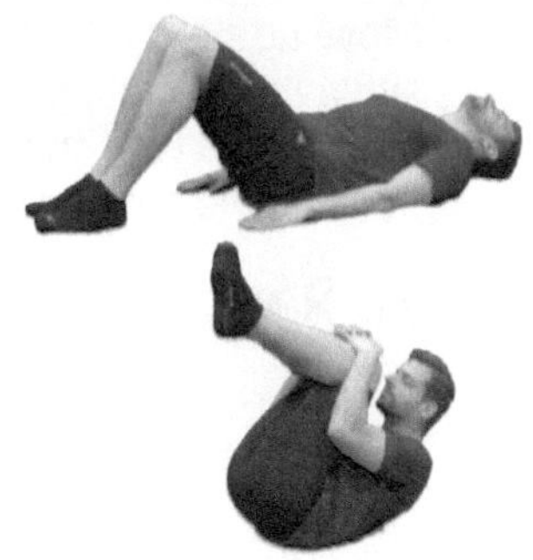

Name: **Quick Wiper |** Time: **7 Minutes**
Type: **Strength** | Level: **Intermediate**
Goal: **Strength** | Intensity: **70%**

(1) Jumping Jacks

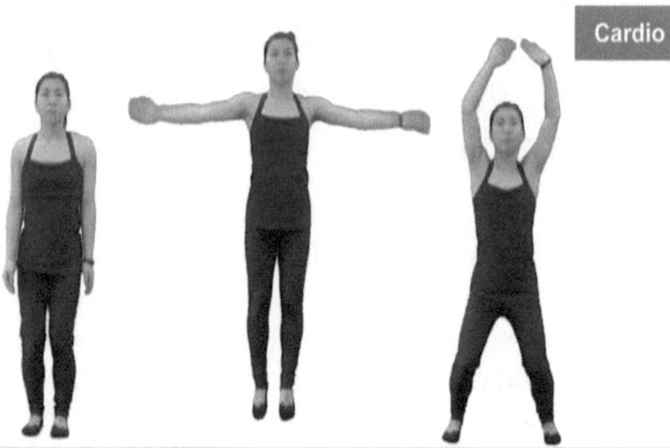

Jump into the air and simultaniously swing your arms up and spread your legs apart. Jump back up to return to the starting position.

60 Seconds

(2) Fly Jacks

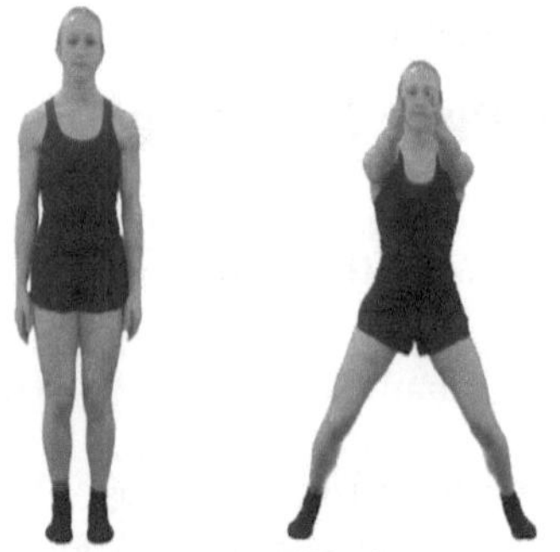

Jump up, swing your arms straight up and spread your legs apart. Jump back up to return to the starting position.

60 Seconds

(3) Get Ups

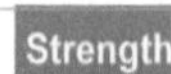

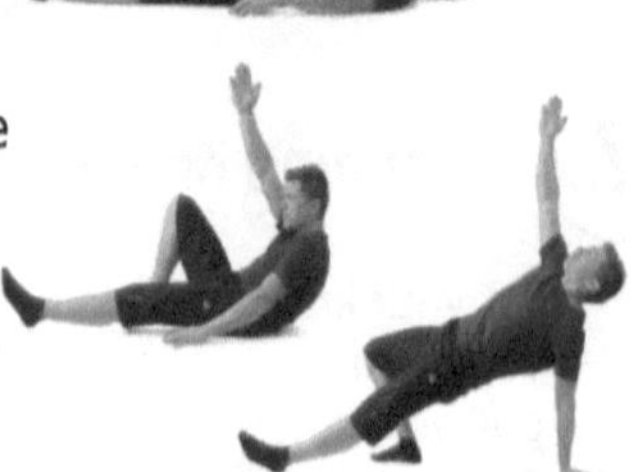

Lie flat on the ground with one knee bent. Move up slowly extending one arm into the air while positioning the other hand underneath your shoulder. Push your hips up and hold for a couple seconds.

10 Reps (per side)

 **Side Vs**

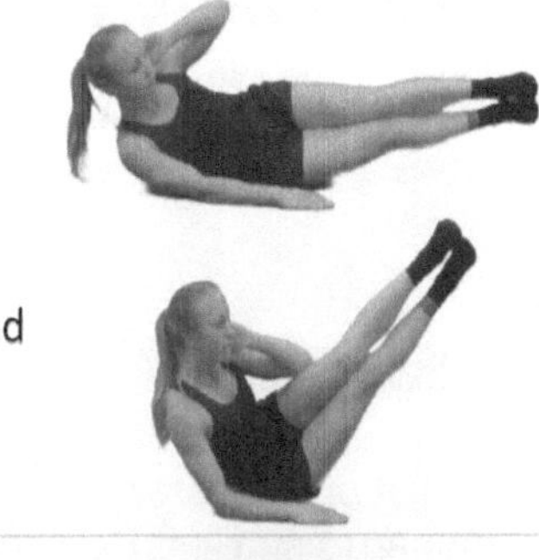

Lie on your side with the hand on top behind your head. Lift your legs straight into the air and move your elbow toward your knees while keeping your hand behind your head.

10 Reps (per side)

 **Jack Knives**

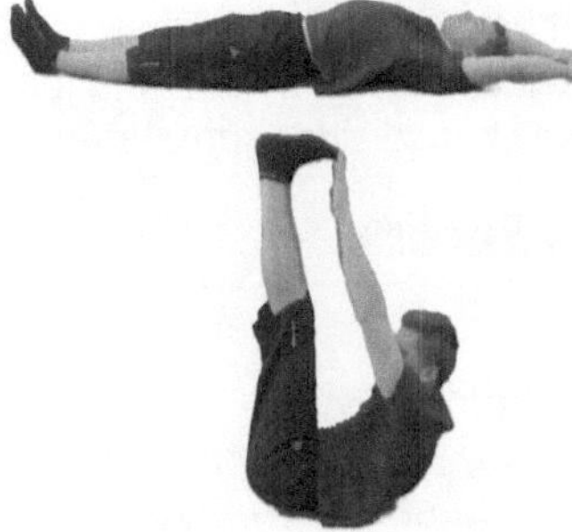

Lie flat on the ground with your arms and legs extended. Lift your arms and legs up, keeping them straight the entire time. Touch your toes at the top. .

20 Reps

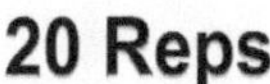

 **Half Wipers**

Flexibility

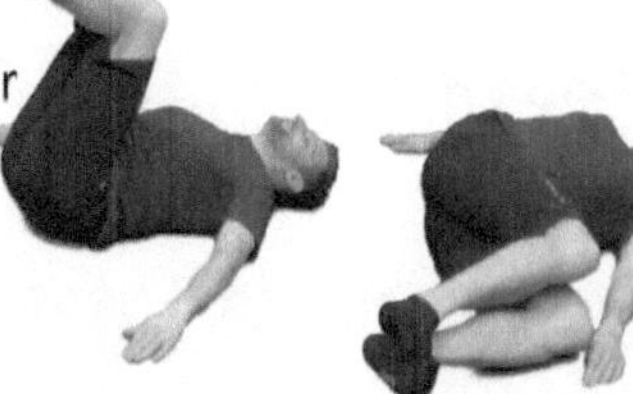

Lay on the ground with your knees bent and your legs lifted into the air. Move your arms to your side with your palms flat on the ground. Keep your shoulders on the ground the entire time.

4x15 Seconds

 **Side Quad Stretch**

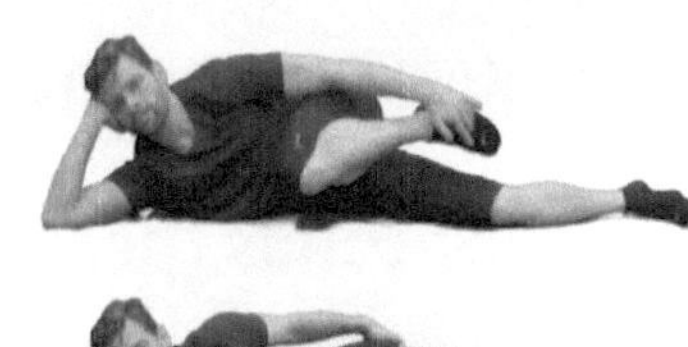

Lay on your side holding on to the ankle of your upper leg. Press your hip forward and pull the foot of the bent leg toward your lower back without shifting your hips.

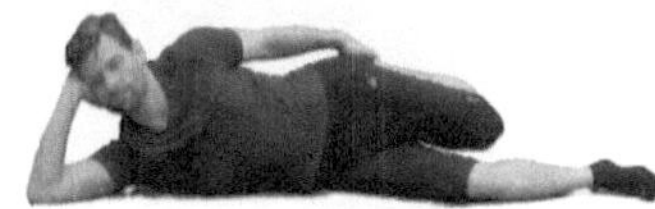

2x30 Seconds

Name: **On Point |** Time: **7 Minutes**
Type: **Flexibility | Level: Beginner**
Goal: **Flexibility | Intensity: 30%**

(1) Swimmer

Strength

Lay flat on your stomach with
your arms and legs extended.
Lift your arms and legs off the ground.
Elevate your right arm and left leg
and change sides simultaniously.

60 Seconds

(2) Child's Pose

Flexibility

Sit on your heals with your
arms by your side. Slowly move
forward with your upper body
extending your arms
as far as possible.

2x30 Seconds

(3) One-legged Pigeon Pose

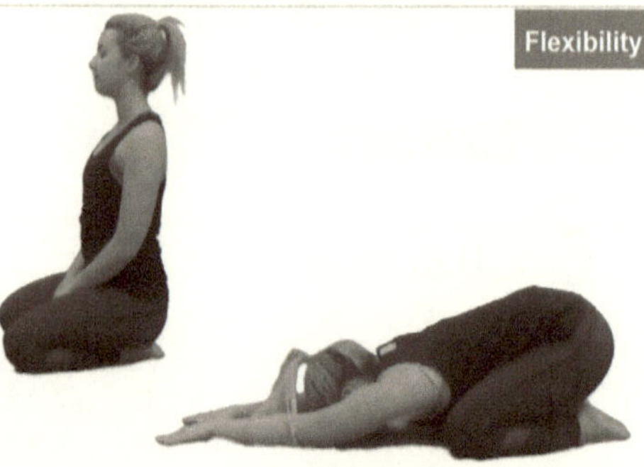

Position your front knee underneath your pecs,
lower the hips toward the ground and straighten
the back leg. Push your upper body upward with
your hands and hold the position.

30 Seconds (per side)

4 — Supine Pigeon Pose

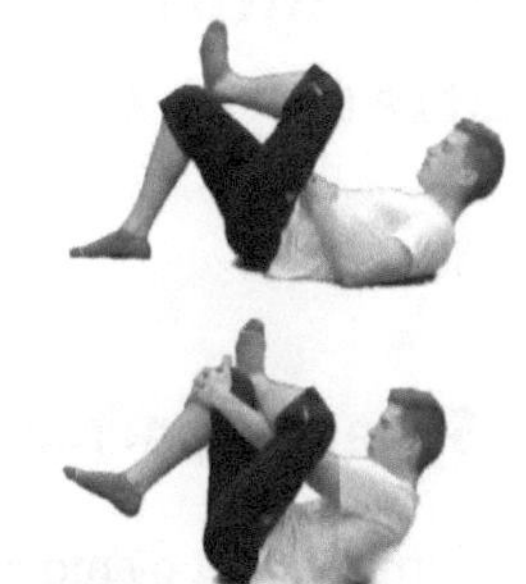

Rest the ankle of the other foot on your quads. Reach with your arms around the knee of the leg that is on the ground and pull it toward your pecs.

30 Seconds (per side)

5 — Toe Stand

Position one leg over the other standing on your toes. Lean forward with your body to increase the stretch in your hip flexors.

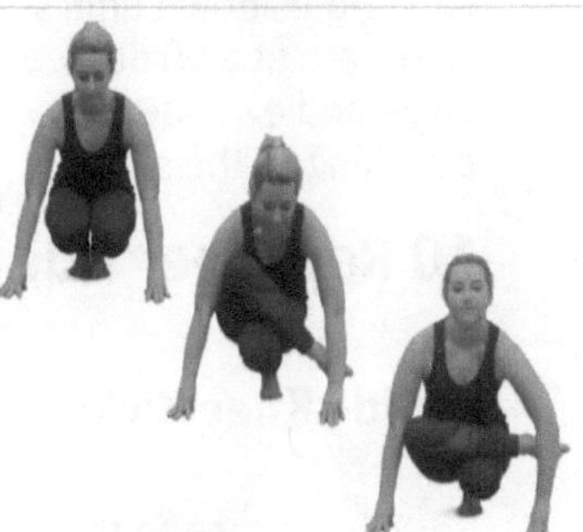

30 Seconds (per side)

6 — Bridge Pose

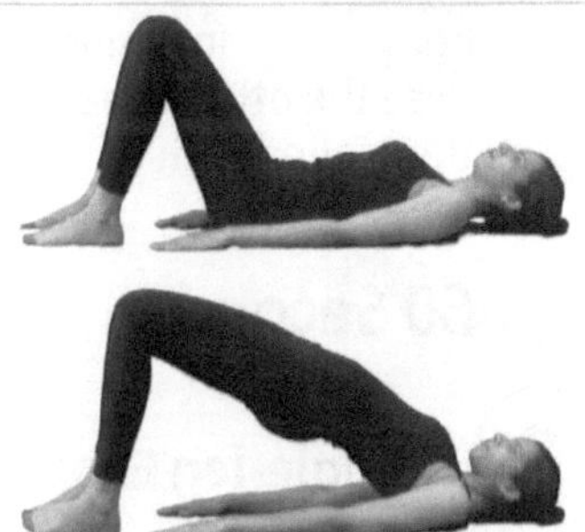

Raise your hips as high as possible and lengthen your lower back. Push your pecs out and hold the position.

2x30 Seconds

7 — Downward-Facing Dog

Lift your hips into the air, extending your arms and legs to create an inverted V shape with your body. Move your pecs toward your legs, lower your body slowly to the starting position.

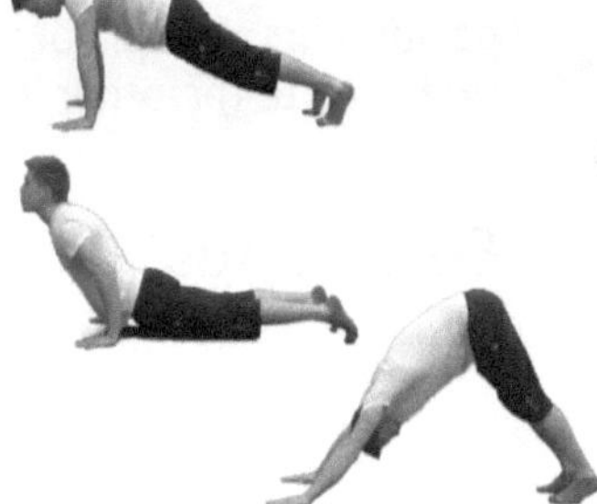

60 Seconds

Name: **Army Style |** Time: **7 Minutes**
Type: **Strength |** Level: **Intermediate**
Goal: **Strength, Physique |** Intensity: **60%**

(1) Squat & Uppercut

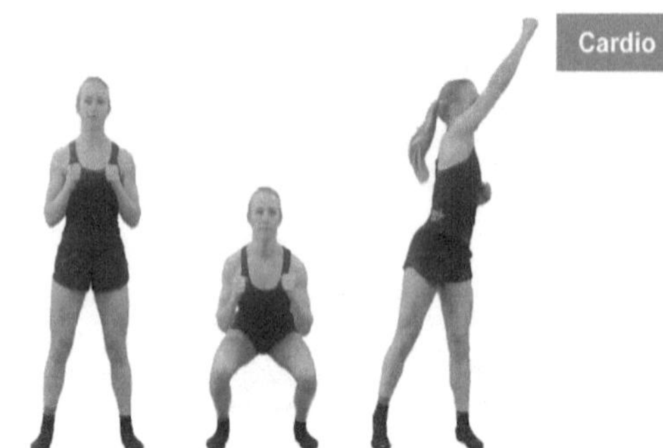

Perform a squat by moving your glutes down until your knees are at a 90 degree angle and explode upward punching to the side.

10 Reps (per side)

(2) Side Knee Kicks

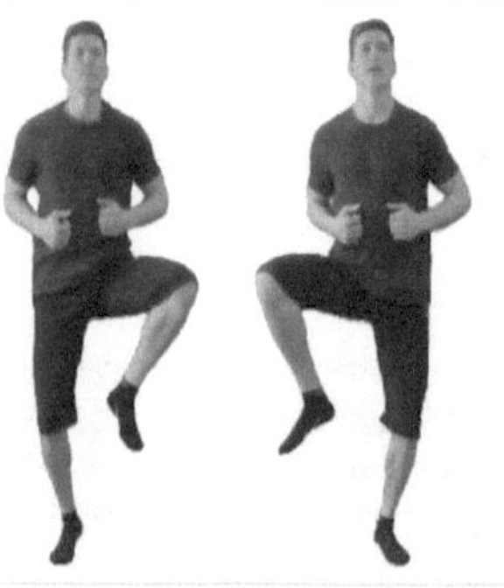

Raise your knee to the side of your body. While lowering the leg in the air raise the other knee, never touching the ground with both feet at the same time.

60 Seconds

(3) Single-leg Elevated Fett Plank

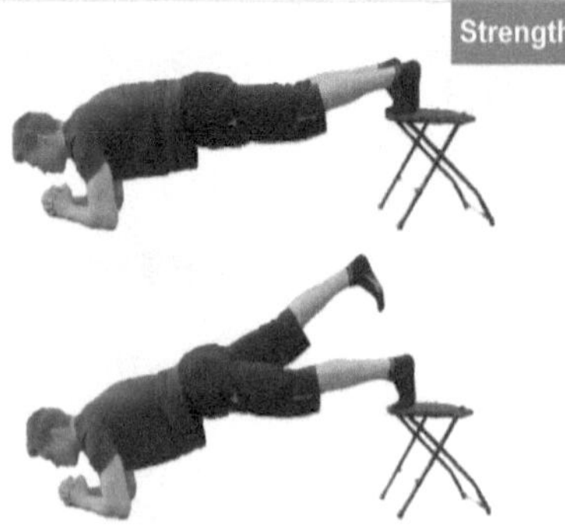

Perform a plank with your feet on a chair. Raise one foot in the air and hold the position for a couple of seconds before switching to the other leg.

60 Seconds

(4) Single-leg Hip Raises

Place the heels of your feet on an elevated suraface. Raise your hips into the air and extend one leg straight into the air. Hold the position at the top for a second and repeat on the same side.

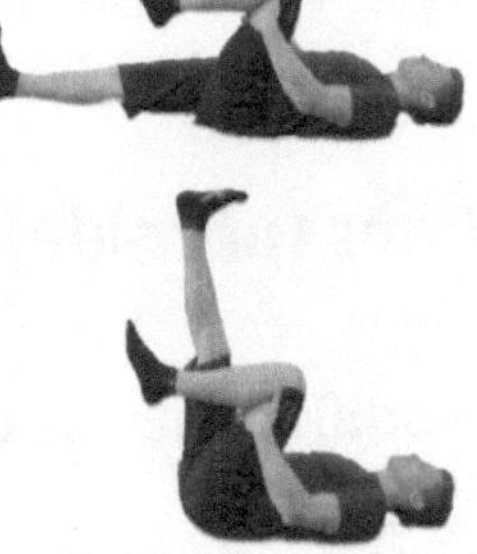

10 Reps (per side)

(5) Single-leg Lowering Drill

Pull your knee toward your chest holding on to the hamstring. Raise the opposite leg straight into the air. Lower the leg slowly without letting the foot touch the ground and repeat on the same side.

10 Reps (per side)

(6) One-legged Hip-opener Squat

Lower your glutes toward the ground with the calve resting on your quad. Raise your arms out straight in front of you and lower your body until your knee is at 90 degrees and stop for a second and push back up.

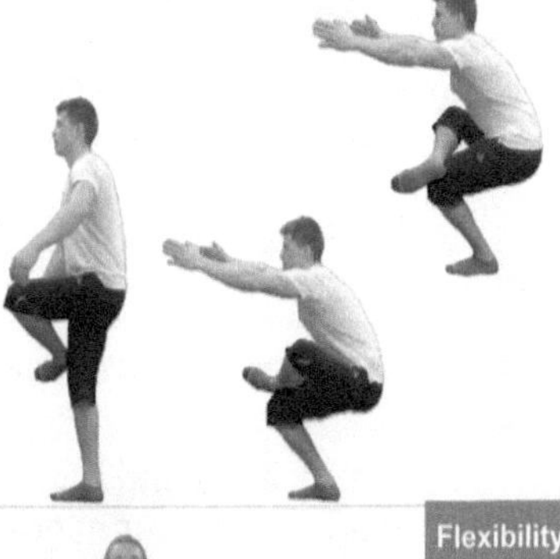

5 Reps (per side)

Flexibility

(7) Wide-legged Forward Bend I

Interlace the fingers of your hands behind your back while upright. Hinge forward from your hips and lower your upper body toward the floor, pulling your interlocked hands toward the floor.

2x30 Seconds

Name: **Anti-Gravity |** Time: **7 Minutes**

Type: Strength | Level: Intermediate

Goal: Strength | Intensity: 60%

(1) Dragon Pushup

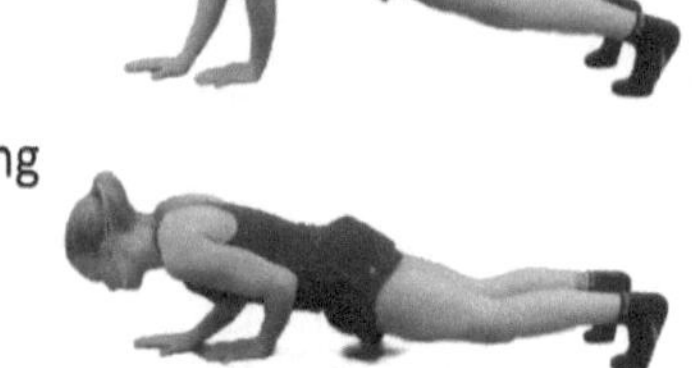

Get into a pushup position, placing one hand above the other. Keep both elbows tucked into your waist, while lowering your body. Repeat in the same position before switching order of hands.

5 Reps (per side)

(2) Modified Diamond Pushup

Get into a pushup position with your knees on the ground and your index fingers and thumbs touching. Lower your body toward the ground and push yourself up forcefully, keeping your elbows bent at the top position.

10 Reps

(3) Lunge with Reverse Fly

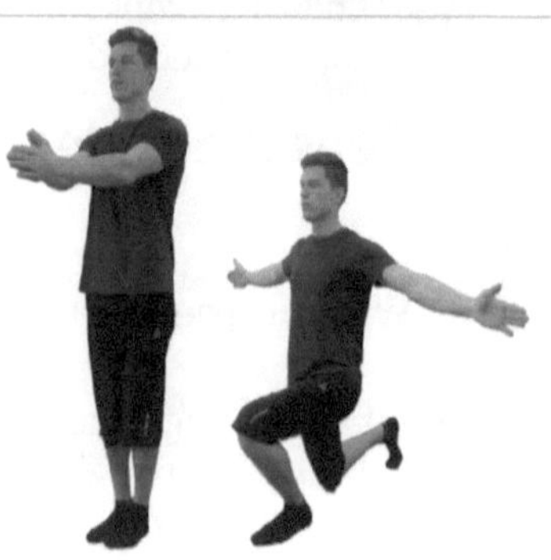

Step back and bend both knees. Open your arms and your hands back as far as possible, keeping both arms straight. Push off with your front foot to move back into the starting position.

10 Reps (per side)

4 Squat Variation

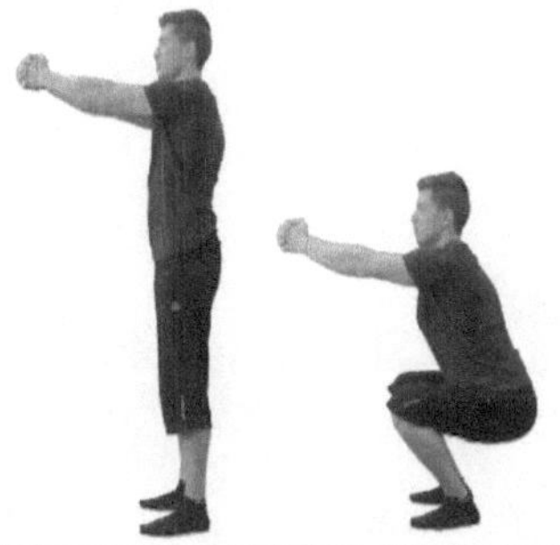

Lower your body until your thighs are parallel to the floor, while keeping your hands interlocked in front. Hold for a second and return to the starting position.

10 Reps (per side)

5 Side Lunges

Take a large step to the side and bend your knee no more than 90 degrees. Explode back to the starting position and switch.

10 Reps (per side)

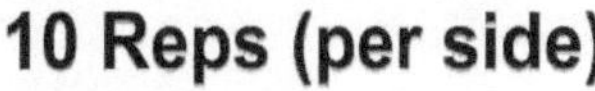

Flexibility

6 The Straddle

Sit on the floor and spread your legs apart. Slowly hinge forward from your hips and move your chest toward the floor.

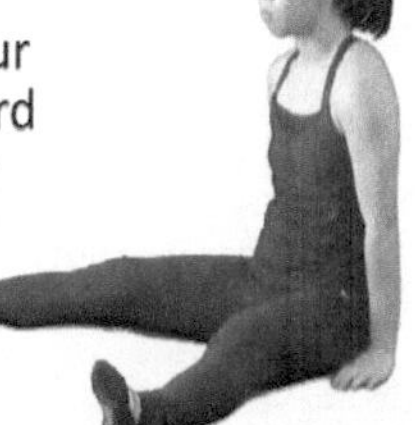

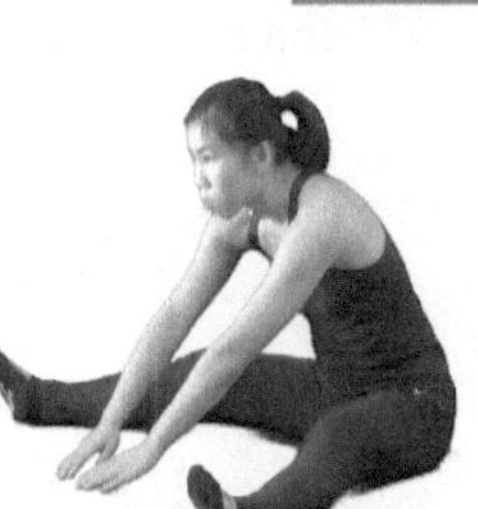

2x30 Seconds

7 Iron Crosses

Lay flat on the ground and move your left leg behind your body to the opposite side. Keep both shoulders on the ground and repeat with the other foot.

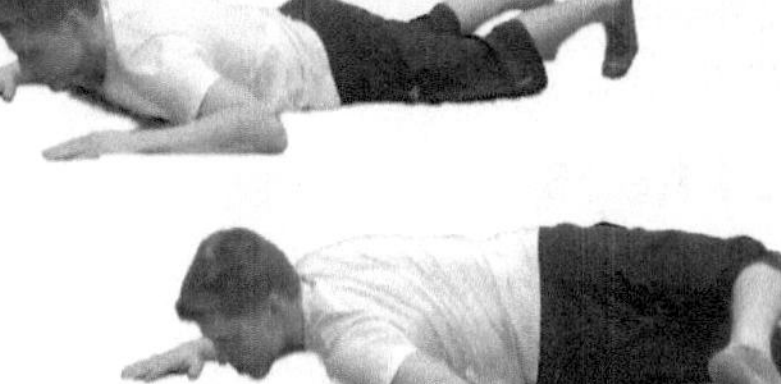

60 Seconds

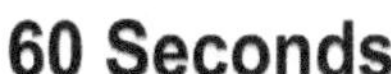

Name: **Chair Master |** Time: **7 Minutes**

Type: **Strength** | Level: **Intermediate**
Goal: **Strength, Stamina** | Intensity: **60%**

(1) Standing Leg Curl

Raise one foot behind you toward your glutes. Hold at the top and tense the muscle in your elevated leg and move back down.

20 Reps (per leg)

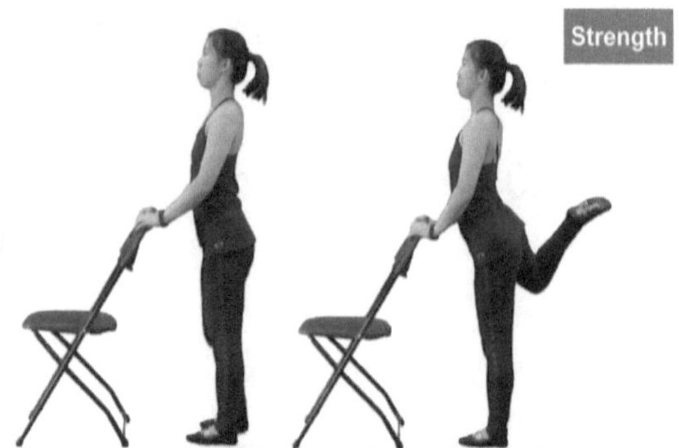

(2) Side Hip Raises

Lift one leg to your side, keeping your pelvis in the same position. Hold the top position briefly and lower your leg to repeat with the same leg.

20 Reps (per leg)

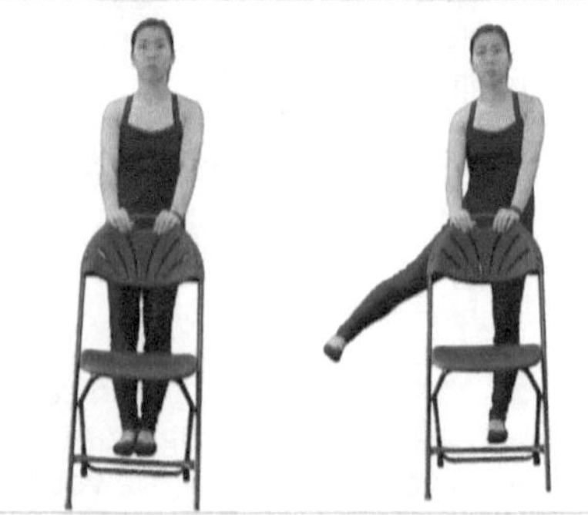

(3) Chair Squats

Interlock your hands and lower your hips until they begin to brush against the chair. Push your hips forward and straighten your legs.

10 Reps

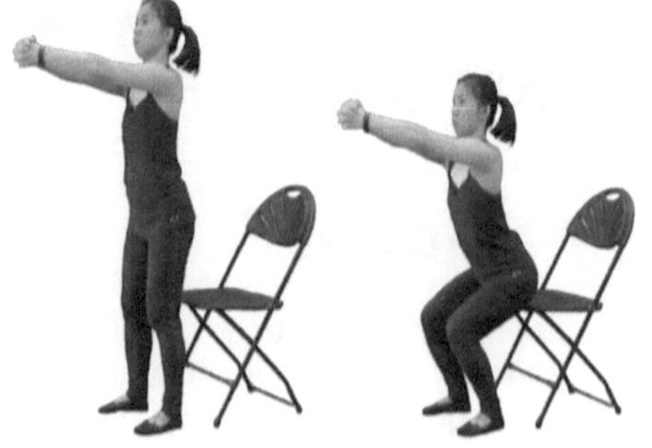

4 Chair Dip

Bend your elbows and lower
your glutes toward the
ground. Gaze forward and
keep your elbows pointing
back.

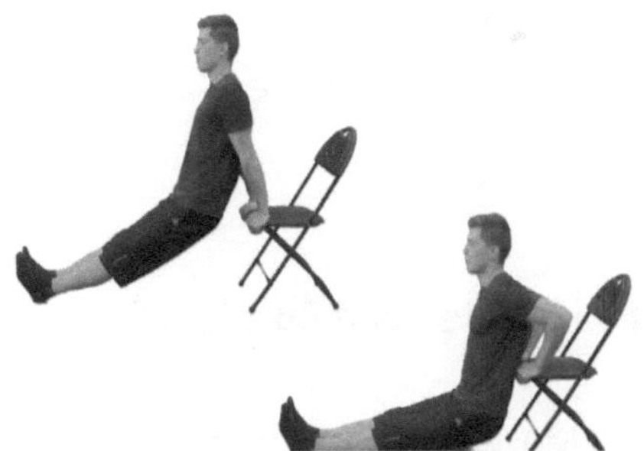

10 Reps

5 Knee Pull-ins

Sit upright and hold on to the side of
the chair to maintain stability. Extend
your legs in front of you, pull your knees toward
your pecs and move them back to
the starting position.

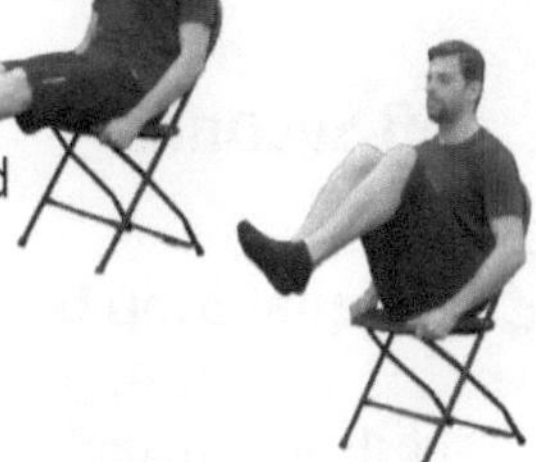

20 Reps

6 Raised Arm Twists

Rotate your body from side to side
keepingyour legs extended in the
same position. To increase the rotation
of your body, lower your hands slightly
during every twist.

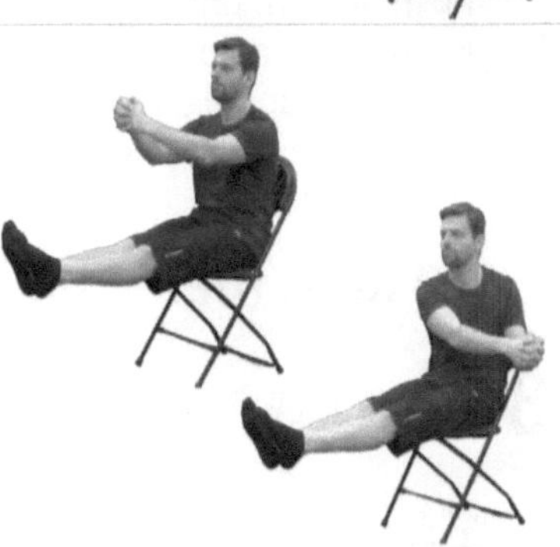

2x30 Seconds

7 Single-leg Bench Get-up

Lower your body without leaning
forward. Gently touch the chair with
your glutes and return to the starting
position. Repeat on the same side with
your arms and leg lifted.

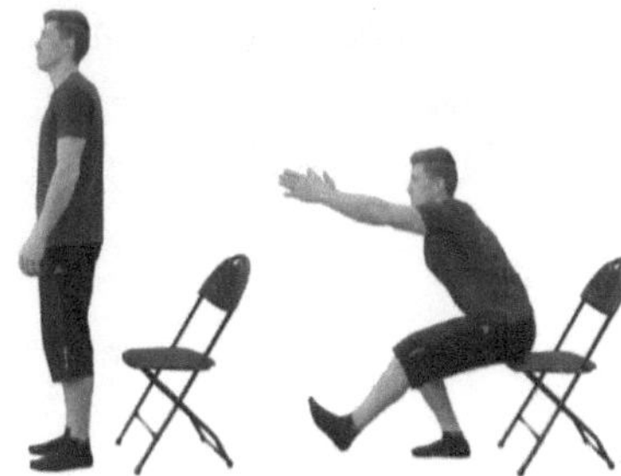

5 Reps (per side)

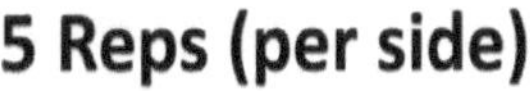

Name: **Lung Test** | Time: **7 Minutes**

Type: **Cardio** | Level: **Beginner**
Goal: **Endurance** | Intensity: **40%**

(1) **Wide Knee Butt kicks**

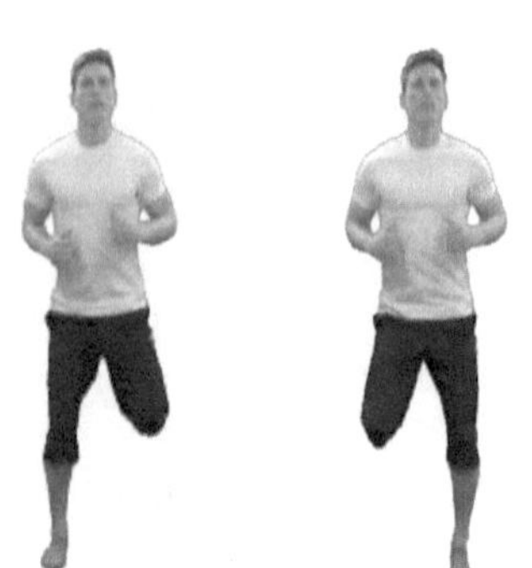

Move in one spot with your legs wider than shoulder-width apart. Lift your heels towards your glutes.

60 Seconds

(2) **Squat Step Ups**

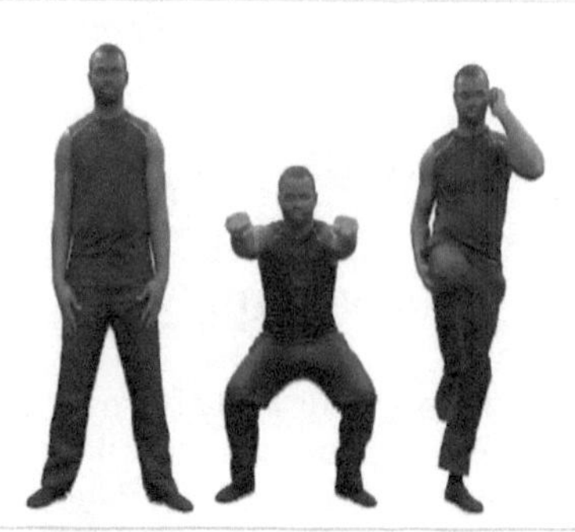

Push up with both legs and raise one knee and the opposite arm halfway through standing. Lower your body back into a squat and repeat on the other side.

10 Reps (per side)

(3) **Side Jacks**

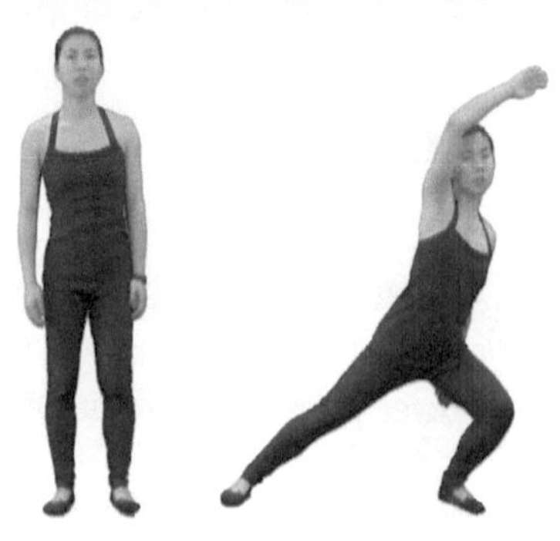

Take a big step to the side, while reaching over your head with your arm.

60 Seconds

 **March Twists**

Interlock your hands in front of your face. Raise your right knee and move your opposite elbow toward the raised knee. Move back down and repeat with the other side.

60 Seconds

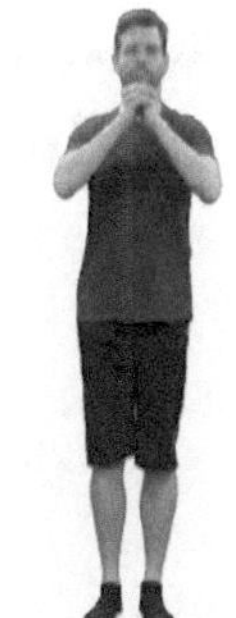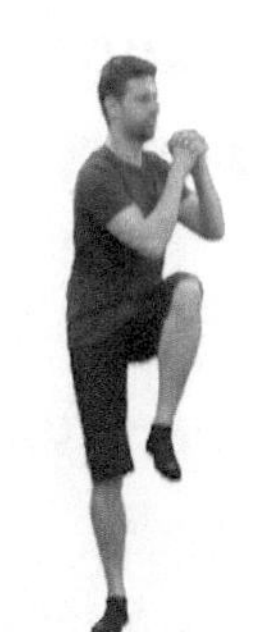

 **Fly Jacks**

Jump up, swing your arms straight up and spread your legs apart. Jump back up to return to the starting position.

60 Seconds

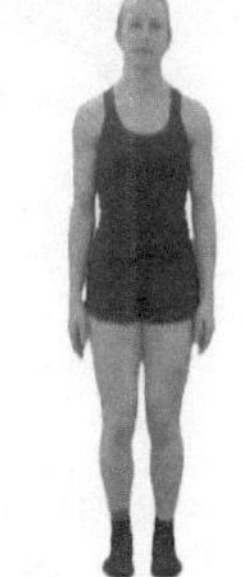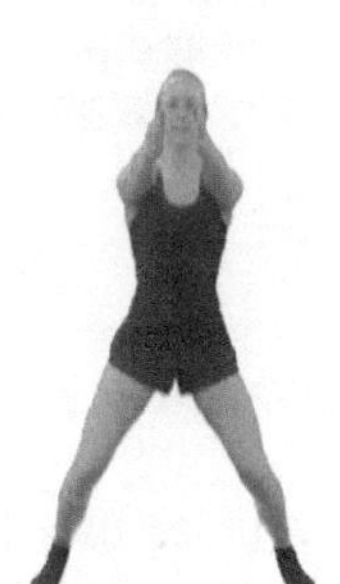

 **Squat Thrusts**

Kick your leg back to land in a pushup position. Bring your legs forward and stand up to repeat the movement.

60 Seconds

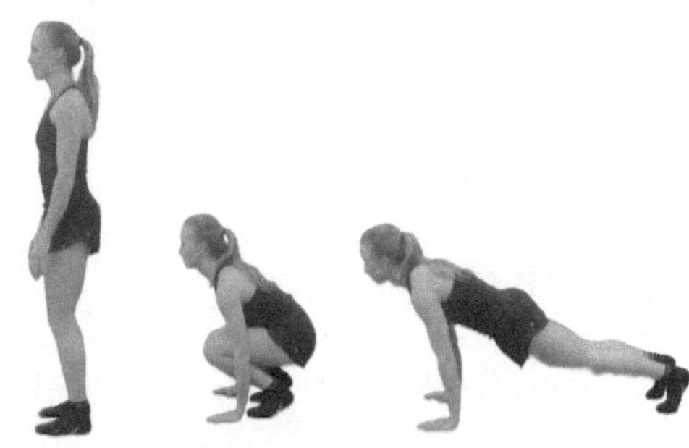

 **Mountain Climbers**

Lift your knee toward your elbow and return your foot to the starting position to repeat with your other leg.

60 Seconds

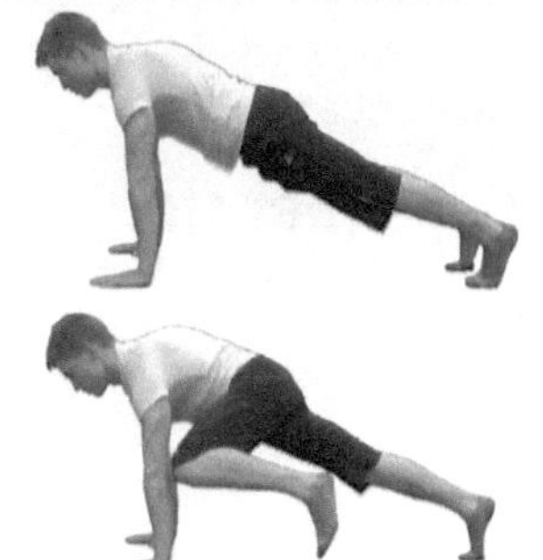

Name: **Final Destination** | Time: **7 Minutes**
Type: **Strength, Flexibility** | Level: **Beginner**
Goal: **Strength, Flexibility** | Intensity: **40%**

---

(1)   **Sitting Punches**

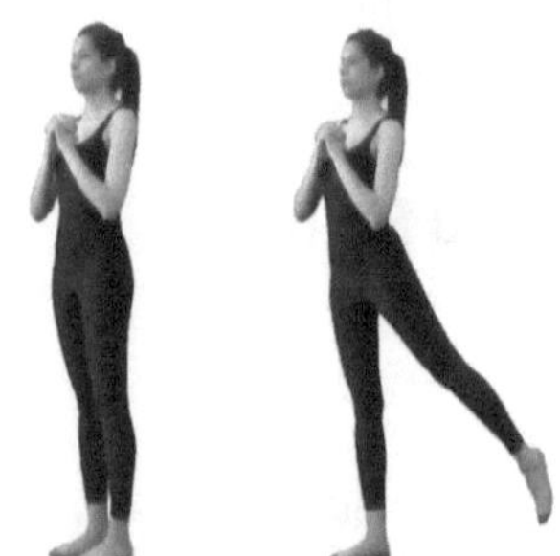

Sit on the floor with your feet off the ground and knees bent. Keep your arms in a boxing position and punch with one arm at a time.

60 Seconds

---

(2)   **Low Back Kicks**

Lift your leg back behind your body and keep it straight. Hold your leg in position for a brief second and slowly lower it to the starting position to repeat with the other leg.

10 Reps (per side)

---

(3)   **Single-leg Squat**

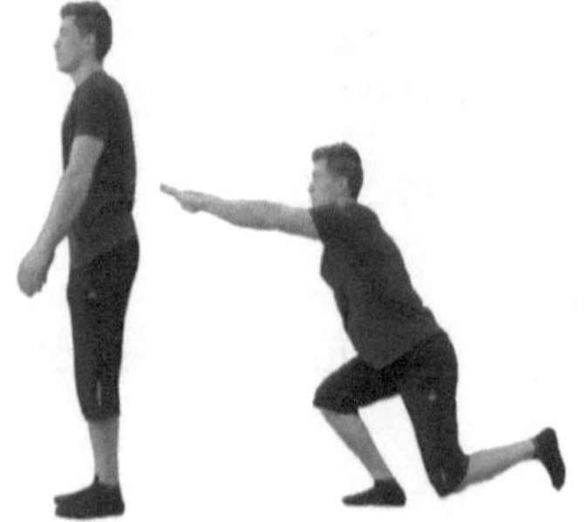

Squat down with one leg, while extending your arms infront. Bend the knee of the front foot no less than 90 degrees. Lift your body back up, keeping your arms in front and repeat.

10 Reps (per side)

(4) Standing Quad Stretch

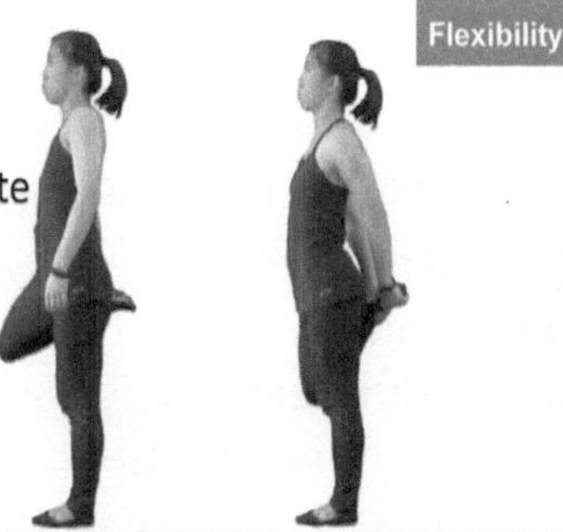

Pull your ankle back as you move the opposite arm toward the other hand for support. Push your hips forward to stretch your quads and thighs.

30 Seconds (per side)

(5) Standing One-legged Ham Stretch

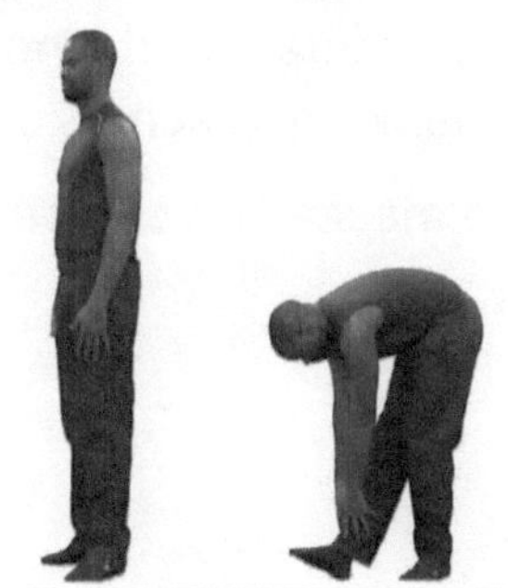

Position one foot in front of the other, bend your back leg and raise your toes. Lean forward and keep the front leg straight.

30 Seconds (per side)

(6) Supine Pigeon Pose

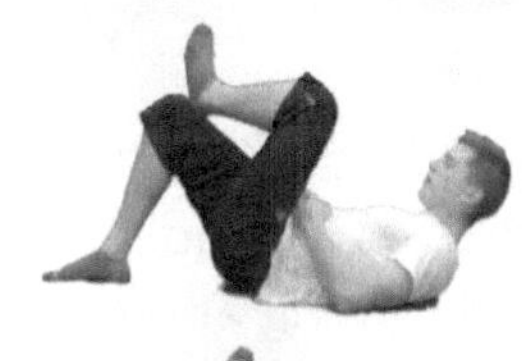

Rest the ankle of the other foot on your quads. Reach with your arms around the knee of the leg that is on the ground and pull it toward your pecs.

30 Seconds (per side)

(7) Low Lunge

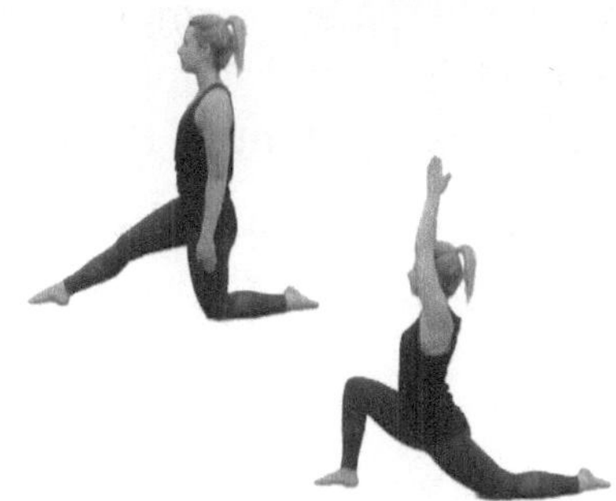

Get into a lunge position, and lean forward with you upper body. Extend your arms over your head and move your hips towards the ground.

2x15 Seconds (per side)

Acknowledgment

I want to thank everyone who has inspired me to live a healthy life and has helped me advance my understanding of my body, my mind, and my eating habits. I am grateful for my parents who enrolled me in countless physical activities as a child and have shared their backgrounds as former professional athletes, physiologists, coaches, and fitness instructors. I thank my friends who have motivated me on tough days and who have helped me stay resilient. Lastly, I want to thank my teachers and mentors for their support over the years to help me stay on course to write this book.

About Author

Noah Kanyo is a former professional athlete, fitness fanatic and jack of all trades, with experience as a personal trainer, and as a swimming and basketball coach. He finished his master's in Physical Education, Kinesiology and Recreation from the University of Alberta and has spent countless hours practicing and learning more about, Yoga, Pilates, Aerobics, Boxing, and Kickboxing. His degree in psychology has helped him recognize the importance of the mind and the vital role it plays in improving the quality of our lives. One of his goals in life is to find simple and effective ways that allow everyone to maximize their potential. He will continue to learn and share his view to inspire others to live a healthy and fulfilling lifestyle.

Also Available from Noah Kanyo:

A comprehensive guide to learn everything about bodyweight fitness.

The Bodyweight Manual Workout

Now available on Amazon.

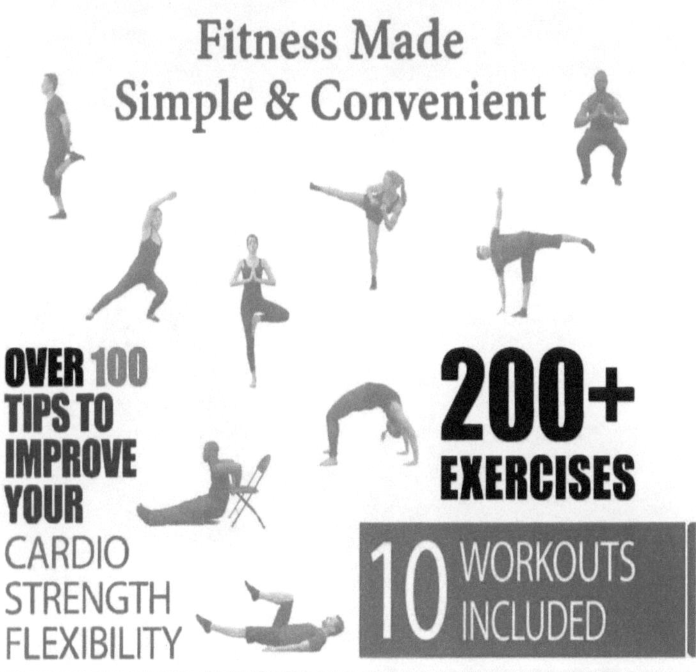